D0017937

dohan

A DOCTOR'S GUIDE TO THERAPEUTIC TOUCH

Most Perigee Books are available at special quantity discounts for bulk purchases for sales promotions, premiums, fund-raising or educational use. Special books, or book excerpts, can also be created to fit specific needs.

For details, write: Special Markets, The Berkley Publishing Group, 200 Madison Avenue, New York, NY 10016.

A DOCTOR'S GUIDE TO THERAPEUTIC TOUCH

Susan Wager, M.D.

Introduction by Dora Kunz

A Perigee Book

Notice: The information in this book is true and complete
to the best of our knowledge. It is not intended as a
replacement for sound medical advice from a doctor.
Important decisions about treating an ill person must be
made by individuals and their doctors. All recommendations
herein are made without guarantees on the part of the
author or the publisher. The author and publisher disclaim
all liability in connection with the use of this information.

A Perigee Book
Published by The Berkley Publishing Group
200 Madison Avenue
New York, NY 10016

Copyright © 1996 by Susan Wager, M.D.
Introduction copyright © 1996 by Dora Kunz
Book design by Rhea Braunstein
Cover design by Dale Fiorillo
Cover and interior illustrations by Daniel Thomas Doolin

All rights reserved. This book, or parts thereof, may not be
reproduced in any form without permission.

First edition: November 1996

Published simultaneously in Canada.

The Putnam Berkley World Wide Web site address is
http://www.berkley.com/berkley

Library of Congress Cataloging-in-Publication Data
Wager, Susan.
    A doctor's guide to therapeutic touch / Susan Wager ;
introduction by Dora Kunz.—1st ed.
        p.   cm.
    "A Perigee book."
    Includes bibliographical references.
    ISBN 0-399-52250-6
    1. Touch—Therapeutic use.   2. Imposition of hands—
Therapeutic use.   3. Vital force—Therapeutic use.
    I. Title.
RZ999.W34   1996
615.8'52—dc20   96-7240
                                        CIP

Printed in the United States of America

10   9   8   7   6   5   4   3   2   1

contents

Introduction

SINCE OUR DEVELOPMENT of Therapeutic Touch in the 1970s, its use has become widespread throughout the United States and Canada. In the East and Midwest particularly, it is taught in nursing schools and practiced in many hospitals. It has also become well-accepted in Canada, especially in Ontario.

Before I developed Therapeutic Touch, I had worked for many years with the medical profession. In the 1930s I began to collaborate with Dr. Otelia Bengtsson, a New York City allergist, using some of my special abilities to understand the relationship between a person's emotions, thought patterns, and their physical illness. Later, at the request of a group of physicians, I observed several famous healers at work. These observations took place over the course of several years, and gave me the opportunity to see people with many different kinds of illness, who were treated with different healing techniques. There were always doctors present to evaluate the effectiveness of the healing. Almost all of the healers I observed were very religious, and stressed the religious aspect of what they were doing to help their patients. Some of the doctors brought their patients to see the healers. The physicians were interested in what the healers were doing to help their patients, but did not usually share the religious interest of the healers.

Because I was born in Indonesia of Dutch parents, and later lived in Australia, the United States, and India, I had the opportunity to observe healing practices in many different cultures. I felt very strongly that healing was a natural potential that human beings could develop, and that it was not dependent on specific religious beliefs.

In the early 1970s I began to develop Therapeutic Touch, in conjunction with Dr. Dolores Krieger, then a professor of Nursing at New York University. I felt at the time that if we could devise a technique, based on our observation of healers, and teach it to health professionals, that many people could be helped. Because Dr. Krieger was a professor of Nursing, we began by teaching Therapeutic Touch to a few of her students. I believed that nurses were good candidates to learn Therapeutic Touch because they were open to the idea of healing. In addition, their technical training gave them some basis for understanding whether or not their use of Therapeutic Touch was effective. I also felt that health professionals could be trained to use this healing technique because they have a sense of compassion for the sick, and a desire to help others. Equally important, I believed that health professionals would take a scientific and realistic approach to Therapeutic Touch, so that we could begin to gather reliable information about its effects.

Therapeutic Touch is based on the ideas that there is a universal healing energy available to all living things, and that we live in an orderly universe. During Therapeutic Touch, the nurses project the idea of healing, and this helps the body to function as a whole, in an orderly way. Over the past twenty-three years we have begun to understand the benefits of Therapeutic Touch. Almost always, Therapeutic

Touch will calm patients and reduce pain. Therapeutic Touch gives sick people more energy so that they can carry on, despite having an illness. It also improves self-confidence: Those who receive Therapeutic Touch often come to feel that they have an inner self that is a source of strength and intuition. This helps a sick person to live to his or her fullest ability despite the presence of disease. Although he may be physically limited, psychologically he can reach out to others and make a contribution.

Besides affecting its recipients, Therapeutic Touch also helps the practitioners. We have observed that nurses and other health professionals who practice Therapeutic Touch develop greater confidence in their ability to help their patients. Besides using their usual medical skills, the practitioners have another way to reduce the anxiety and pain of their patients. Therapeutic Touch practitioners also learn to keep their minds and emotions quiet. This helps transmit a sense of peace to their patients, and also keeps the health professionals from getting emotionally disturbed by the problems of their patients.

There is now far more acceptance of Therapeutic Touch in medical settings than there was when we started it. People are more aware that there are other ways of healing besides conventional medicine, and that the sick can sometimes be helped by simple methods. Even so, I feel strongly that we stick to scientific standards in evaluating Therapeutic Touch and its effects, and that it be considered an addition to conventional medical care, not a replacement for it. I would therefore like to see Therapeutic Touch remain in the province of health professionals, who have the training to assess its usefulness.

In the pages that follow, Dr. Wager explains the ideas behind the development of Therapeutic Touch, and presents some of the existing research on the subject. This scientific

approach is an important one, and adds to the already existing literature on Therapeutic Touch. My hope for the future is that we continue this kind of scientific evaluation,
because it will help us to develop our understanding of the
healing process.

DORA KUNZ

Preface

BEFORE I ATTENDED medical school, I was interested in the philosophy of healing. I was aware of the varied healing practices of many cultures, both ancient and modern. I had heard of spiritual and hands-on healing practices, and had seen a few cases where recipients of healing had improved. I was curious about the *how* of this kind of healing. I could accept the possibility of nontraditional healing, but also believed that there must be underlying rational principles at work that I did not understand.

In July of 1979 I began an internship in Internal Medicine at a major medical center in New York City. For the next three years, I was absorbed in mastering the complex content of medicine, and was preoccupied with the never-ending responsibilities of the medical intern. In this atmosphere, I had no time for philosophical ideas about healing, but instead was involved in the practical aspects of becoming a physician—care of patients, attendance at medical conferences, and simply surviving the many sleepless nights imposed by my responsibilities at a large city hospital.

About halfway through my internship I began to feel that I was living a contradiction. I had chosen a career in medicine to help others, but as the medical intern, I had become the agent of pain, discomfort, or inconvenience to my patients. I had the responsibility for drawing their blood, probing their wounds, waking them in the middle of the night to restart intravenous lines, and announcing the next uncomfortable test or procedure that was awaiting them. I wondered if there wasn't a better way to treat the sick.

At the same time, I saw most of my patients, and those of my colleagues, improve as a result of their medical care. I learned that the application of science and medical technology could improve health and relieve suffering. As I became a more skilled physician, I experienced the rewards of using my hands and my mind to help others. Despite this, there was still something missing. As my fellow residents and I became more adept at solving the problems of our patients, we became more removed from them as people. This happened not because we were uncaring, but because the pressures of a busy routine on the hospital ward left very little time for anything else except a scientific consideration of the disease process and its remedies. In addition, as we developed our analytic skills, we often disregarded our intuitive abilities, sometimes to the detriment of the patient.

In 1982, at the end of my medical residency, I attended a conference on healing in Washington, D.C. I was there at the suggestion of my sister, Kathleen, a music therapist. At the time, the idea of attending a meeting about healing was not terribly appealing to me. As a busy physician, I preferred to think about anything other than sickness when I had a chance to be away from the hospital. Nevertheless, I agreed to go, mostly because the meeting gave me an opportunity to visit my sister, who lived in another city.

At the conference I was amazed to find more than a thousand people from a variety of health professions who had gathered to discuss both methods and philosophies of healing. One of the participants was Dr. Dolores Krieger, an originator of Therapeutic Touch. She gave a short presentation about Therapeutic Touch, and then demonstrated the technique. I was interested and intrigued, both by the sense of peace that descended in the room when Dr. Krieger began her treatment, and the apparent feeling of well-being that her patient experienced.

On my return to New York, I sought Therapeutic Touch training. Because Dr. Krieger was a professor of Nursing at New York University, its graduate school of nursing offered training in Therapeutic Touch, and I attended classes and workshops there. I refined my skills by practicing on friends, family, and other students of the technique, and at the same time, I continued my medical practice. Because of its unconventional nature, I did not use Therapeutic Touch in the care of my patients at the time.

In 1984, I met Dora Kunz, the other originator of Therapeutic Touch. Over the course of a few days, at a conference in Boston, I observed her treating patients with Therapeutic Touch. Some of the people she saw were very seriously ill, and had been sent to her by physicians who knew of her work. Others had less severe illness. I noticed that most patients treated by Dora experienced relief of pain and a reduction in their anxiety. Sometimes seriously ill patients, who were fearful of the prospect of suffering until death, were relieved of their discomfort and fear of the unknown. When I subsequently had opportunities to observe Dolores Krieger at work, or the advanced practitioners she had trained, I noted that their patients had the same beneficial results.

As a physician who values the scientific method, I approached Therapeutic Touch with openness, yet also with a healthy skepticism. I was wary of nontraditional techniques that promised more than they could deliver, or took advantage of a desperate patient's need to be well. What I found with Therapeutic Touch was an approach that was modest in its claims. Its originators were very clear that Therapeutic

Touch was not a replacement for regular medical care, but should be used as an adjunct. Although Therapeutic Touch did seem to stimulate the body's natural healing process, its practitioners did not promise to cure the underlying disease of the patient, or even that his symptoms would necessarily improve. They pointed out that the most common experience of patients was reduction in pain and relaxation, and even if Therapeutic Touch produced no other benefits, that these results would be worthwhile. Both Dora Kunz and Dolores Krieger, as well as the nurses they had trained, always encouraged their patients to continue their usual medical therapy, and supported their self-help efforts. I was impressed by this commonsense approach and continued to study Therapeutic Touch and its effects.

From my perspective, the most striking result of Therapeutic Touch was that almost every patient treated felt a sense of well-being, and often a peace of mind that was not present before treatment. Although medical cure eluded many seriously ill people, their suffering was at least partially relieved. Whether or not the sick people improved physically, they often experienced a surge of vitality and creativity, which allowed them to lead more productive lives, despite their disabilities. The patients experienced themselves as making a contribution to their families or society, and having an identity greater than their illness.

One patient's story illustrates this:

A woman in her forties, whom I will call Jane, had multiple sclerosis. This disease affects the lining of the nerve cell, called myelin. Over time, small holes develop in the myelin, and the speed with which impulses are conducted through the nerve slows down. As a result, people with multiple sclerosis exhibit a wide variety of symptoms, the most obvious of which is muscle weakness. When Jane came to Dora Kunz for Therapeutic Touch treatments, she had some weakness in her legs. She was able to walk independently most of the time, but sometimes needed crutches to maintain her balance. Over the course of a few years, she received many Therapeutic Touch treatments, in addition to her usual medical therapies. Despite this, she continued to deteriorate, and eventually spent more and more time at home. Although her physical condition worsened, she responded creatively. She started her own business at her house, and maintained a great deal of contact with both her business associates and her friends, who came to see her at home.

My impression at the time was that Therapeutic Touch was instrumental in changing her view of herself and her capabilities. Instead of withdrawing because of her illness, she developed the energy and sense of self to live fully, within her physical limitations.

Over the past thirteen years I have treated hundreds of patients with Therapeutic Touch. I have also observed many patients treated by Dora Kunz, Dolores Krieger, and the practitioners they have trained. I continue to be impressed with the ability of Therapeutic Touch to relieve pain and decrease anxiety. In addition, I have noticed that many patients who receive Therapeutic Touch experience faster healing of infections and wounds. I have treated patients with serious illness, such as cancer, HIV disease, and multiple sclerosis, who lived longer with their illnesses than I expected, and were able to enjoy life, despite the presence of serious illness.

Besides helping the recipients, Therapeutic Touch also affects its practitioners. After a few years of practice, most of them become more intuitive and creative. They usually find that their outer life experience reflects more accurately their inner feelings and beliefs. The many nurses and some physicians who practice Therapeutic Touch also find that it fosters a greater sense of emotional connection to their patients. I personally feel more empathy for my patients, but at the same time am less apt to become overidentified with their problems. Most other experienced practitioners report this as well. Perhaps even more important, through the practice of Therapeutic Touch, most practitioners develop a deeper understanding of the relationship between the body, mind, and emotions. We no longer think of disease as affecting only the body, but realize that there is a complex relationship between our physical health and our habitual thoughts and feelings.

Because of its effects on both patients and practitioners, I believe that Therapeutic Touch has a place beside the best that medical technology has to offer in the care of the sick. Very often medical care palliates, but does not cure. If the patient's recovery from illness is not possible, the aim of his physician and nurses is to maximize the quality of life, while minimizing the suffering. Therapeutic Touch provides an opportunity for doing so.

This book provides a basic description of the technique of Therapeutic Touch in a way that I hope the average person can understand. It also explores why it is that Therapeutic Touch promotes healing, and examines the philosophical assumptions on which it is based. These assumptions, as the reader will see, make Therapeutic Touch a natural complement to Western medicine.

At present, Therapeutic Touch is taught in many nursing schools, and practiced in hospitals throughout the country. It has largely been through the pioneering efforts of the nursing profession that Therapeutic Touch has been made available to the sick. A few medical schools have shown some interest in Therapeutic Touch, but as far as I am aware, there are none which include it in their curriculum. It is my hope for the future that Therapeutic Touch be easily integrated into our medical care, and that we continue to increase our understanding of its effects with the scientific approach begun by Dolores Krieger and Dora Kunz.

Acknowledgments

THE CHALLENGE OF producing a book can be daunting to a first-time author. This task was made easier by the gracious help of many.

My thanks to Jacky Olitsky for the early research that got this project rolling, and to Kirsten Van Gelder for generously allowing me access to her personal library. I am also grateful to John Kunz for discussion of his remembrance of the early days of Therapeutic Touch, and for sharing audiotapes which were helpful for background information.

I am indebted to several members of the Nurse Healers Professional Associates, who provided me with useful information about Therapeutic Touch research, valuable suggestions for people to interview, and lots of support and encouragement. Thanks to Sue Wright, Barbara Cull-Wilby, Patricia Winstead Fry, Nelda Samarel, Melodie Olson and Ann Clark.

There were many Therapeutic Touch practitioners who shared their personal experiences with me, some of whom are mentioned in this book. Gary Bachman and George Clark told me of their work caring for the dying. Sally Blumenthal-McGannon contributed not only her knowledge about Therapeutic Touch, but made valuable suggestions based on her counseling experience with the seriously ill, especially her patients suffering from AIDS. Both Joanne O'Reilly and Linda Schill shared their wealth of experience treating infants and children with Therapeutic Touch, and generously reviewed that part of the manuscript. Jane Williams gave me much valuable information on her work with people suffering chronic pain. Sandra Revesz not only lent her considerable expertise in Therapeutic Touch, but provided me with encouragement at every step in the process. She was always available for questions large and small, and I am grateful to count her as one of my friends.

I would also like to thank the patients who were willing to be interviewed for this book. Aside from Jim Schultz, who has done considerable public speaking to help others, they will not be named here in order to preserve their privacy. Their generosity, openness, and honesty has allowed us to understand more about Therapeutic Touch and its effects.

Of course, no book would exist without its editor. I am grateful for John Duff, who had the idea for this book, and believed in my ability to produce it. His advice and encouragement kept this project going, and his flexibility, patience, and insight were remarkable.

There are others who helped with the technical aspects. Dan Doolin's illustrations capture beautifully the spirit of Therapeutic Touch, and his unfailing sense of humor made our collaboration a joy. My sister, Kathleen Wager, graciously read most of the manuscript, making time in her already busy life.

I am most grateful for the personal support provided by friends and family. Petra Ronish deserves special mention for her loving care of my son, which gave me the time I needed to write. My husband, Greg Gottlieb, a fantastic jack-of-all-trades, provided ideas, hours of manuscript reading, and even more hours of child care to support the completion of this project. That he managed to do all this while attending to the demands of a busy medical practice is testimony both to his energy and generosity of spirit.

My last and deepest thank you is to Dora Kunz, whose assistance was both generous and invaluable. Together we spent hours deciding on the content of each chapter, and how best to express the essence of Therapeutic Touch in a way that could be easily understood. She read every page of the manuscript and provided valuable suggestions.

Even more significantly, many of the ideas expressed in this book are the result of Dora's lifelong dedication to helping the sick. For over sixty years, she has had the opportunity to observe the effects of healing practices. Her inquiring and scientific approach enabled her to work out a body of knowledge which she has willingly shared with health professionals, caring only that her ideas be used to help others, and not that she receive specific acknowledgment. Although this book is written through the filter of my experience, her contribution is reflected on many of these pages.

1

Origins

IN THE INTENSIVE care unit of a large hospital, a two-pound premature infant lies, attached to monitors, restless and breathing rapidly. Her nurse appears at the bedside and gently begins to pass her hands over the baby, a few inches from the surface of her skin. While the nurse does this, she becomes calm within, and thinks of the baby as peaceful and comfortable. In a few minutes the baby's rapid respiration slows and she falls asleep.

In the orthopedics clinic of the same hospital, a 26-year-old-man is seeing his physician three weeks after a serious fracture. The doctor is amazed to see that the X ray shows improvement that he would normally expect after six to eight weeks. This patient, since breaking his leg, has been treated twice weekly by a nurse who has gently and rhythmically passed her hands over the fracture, a few inches from his skin. Like the nurse treating the premature baby, this practitioner becomes calm, and while working with the patient, thinks of him as whole and well, and of the fractured bone as completely healthy.

In a medical office, a physician sees a 45-year-old-man with a leg wound, caused by wearing too-tight ski boots for several days. While cleaning and dressing the wound, she visualizes the patient as well, and imagines the skin to be completely healthy. She is surprised to see that three days later the wound is over 70% healed.

These health professionals are practicing a technique called Therapeutic Touch, a method of balancing and increasing the body's energy to promote healing. It is based on the belief that there is, in living beings, a thrust toward order that is inherent in the healing process. Therapeutic Touch is also based on the idea, common to both Eastern and Native American traditions, that the human being is not merely a mind inhabiting a body, but a complex system of energy. Each person has a physical body, and also possesses the ability to feel, to think, and to understand the world in an intuitive way. Therapeutic Touch practitioners think of these human capacities as each associated with its own characteristic kind of energy. Our physical, emotional, mental, and intuitive energies interact continuously. They have a characteristic pattern and rhythm in each individual.

In health, these energies flow freely, and our intuitive, emotional, and mental energy nourishes us physically. In illness, this energy flow partially constricts, and energy exchange with the environment slows down. Therapeutic Touch promotes healing by helping the body, mind, emotions, and intuition to work together, and by increasing the amount of energy available to the sick person.

Therapeutic Touch was developed in the early 1970s by Dr. Dolores Krieger, then a professor of Nursing at New York University, and Dora Kunz, the former President of the Theosophical Society in America. Since its inception Therapeutic Touch has become an integral part of the care that many nurses, and some physicians, provide. Therapeutic Touch is practiced extensively in the United States and to a lesser extent in Europe, Australia, and Africa. Some nursing schools in the United States include courses in Therapeutic

Touch. Many hospitals, as well, offer workshops in the technique to their health professionals.

Dolores Krieger and Dora Kunz developed Therapeutic Touch as an extension of professional skills for those in the health care field. Because most of its practitioners are health professionals, they advocate that patients who receive Therapeutic Touch continue to follow the medical recommendations of their physicians. Therapeutic Touch is practiced as an adjunct to conventional medical care, not as a replacement. Over the past twenty years, the information that practitioners have gathered through clinical experience and research demonstrates that Therapeutic Touch is effective in relieving pain and anxiety, and in speeding the body's normal healing process. Therapeutic Touch promotes the healing of wounds, fractures, and infections, for example. When nurses treat patients prior to surgery, it shortens their postoperative recovery time. Therapeutic Touch improves breathing in asthmatics and reduces chest pain in emergency room patients. Nurses and physicians have used Therapeutic Touch to comfort the dying and their families. Death is more peaceful for the dying person and the family experiences less anxiety.

Although Therapeutic Touch was developed a little more than twenty years ago, it is based on the ancient practice of laying on of hands. It is fundamentally different from this practice, however, because it is not done in a religious context, and requires no special religious or cultural beliefs on the part of the patient or practitioner. Therapeutic Touch is grounded in the idea that a human being is a system of energy, and that we can direct this energy in a specific way to help one another.

Both Dolores Krieger and Dora Kunz brought unique abilities to the development of Therapeutic Touch. Krieger had a long experience in working with the sick, a solid scientific training, and teaching ability. Kunz, in her late sixties at the time she developed Therapeutic Touch, brought a clear intuitive ability to perceive the disease process in the organs of the body, and to understand how our emotions and thoughts affect the body's health.

Dora Kunz has enhanced her perceptive abilities by lifelong study and careful observation. In the 1930s she began to collaborate with Dr. Otelia Bengtsson, a physician who specialized in allergy and immunology in New York City. She used this opportunity to study carefully the relationships between emotional patterns and physical disease. Since that time she has worked closely with many physicians. Over the past fifty years, she has continued to refine her understanding of the role that emotions and habitual thoughts play in promoting physical illness, and how they facilitate healing.

In the late 1960s a group of physicians invited Dora Kunz to observe several famous healers at work, including Katherine Kuhlman and Ambrose and Olga Worrall. Also among the healers she studied was Oskar Estebany, an unassuming man who had been an Austrian World War I fighter pilot, then later a colonel in the Hungarian cavalry. He discovered his unusual healing abilities while in the military. Colonel Estebany was tending a horse that had been seriously injured one evening. Because the horse was not expected to recover, he feared that the horse would be shot the following morning. He stayed awake through the night, stroking and comforting the horse. To his surprise, the horse was completely well the next day. Other soldiers began to ask Colonel Estebany to care for their animals, and found that he could help many of them. As a result, sick people began to approach him for assistance. Although he was skeptical that he could benefit them, he tried. Again, he succeeded, usually helping sick people to improve at least partially, and sometimes dramatically. One of his patients, a six-year-old girl from Rochester, New York, had an inoperable brain tumor. Oskar Estebany treated her during some clinical studies that both Dora Kunz and Dolores Krieger observed. During the year following the child's initial treatment, Estebany treated her at least twice. After one year, her physicians reported that her brain tumor was undetectable. For at least six years she remained healthy before being lost to follow-up.

Although this case represents vast improvement, most people treated by healers such as Oskar Estebany experience partial improvement, not miracle cures. The healer is probably able to accelerate, at least temporarily, the natural healing processes of the body. From time to time, the results may be as dramatic as those for the six-year-old girl with the brain tumor, but more often the patient's own healing process is set in motion, so that partial improvement, which may be temporary or permanent, can occur.

Because of Dora Kunz's perceptive abilities, during her observations of Colonel Estebany, she noticed the healing energies that he was transmitting, and saw how they affected the body. Colonel Estebany was able to change the disease pattern, and to relieve the pain of his patients. From her observations, both of Estebany and others, she concluded that the ability to heal could be taught. This opinion differed from that of many of the healers she observed, who believed that their abilities were a gift, often tied to their religious or cultural beliefs, and not something others might learn. Because Dora grew up in Indonesia, lived in Australia, and traveled extensively to India and Europe, she had an experience of different cultures that suggested to her that the ability to accelerate healing was not tied to particular cultural or religious beliefs. She believed that some individuals might be better able to heal than others, just as some people were born with more musical talent, for example. Nevertheless, an ability to heal could be taught.

At the time that Dora Kunz was observing the healers, Dr. Dolores Krieger was studying the medical outcome for the patients treated by Colonel Estebany. In a speech which she gave at the Menninger Foundation in 1988,[1] she recounts the following:

My initial interest in healing came through research. In the late sixties, I was asked to take part in some clinical studies on the laying on of hands with which Dora was involved as a finely sensitive observer. My responsibilities were peripheral to the main focus. In retrospect, I realize that these sometimes routine tasks gave me considerable opportunity to exercise strongly skills of observation and inquiry that I had honed as a registered nurse and as a recent Ph.D. The success of the healer, Oskar Estebany, in either ameliorating or removing the symptoms of many of the subjects, who, in medical opinion, either had reached a static plateau in their disease process or who were in the degenerative stages of their illness, surprised and intrigued me. In my experience as a nurse, these types of patients would be lingering in the back wards, once it had been agreed that nothing more could be done for them from a medical perspective.

The success of Colonel Estebany led Dr. Krieger to further study the effects of healing. She found that the available research included studies done on animals and plants, but not on humans. In 1961, Dr. Bernard Grad, a biochemist at McGill University, collaborated with R. V. Cadoret and G. I. Paul to study the effects of the laying on of hands on wound healing in mice.[2] Three hundred mice, each of which had the same size skin wound, were divided randomly into three groups. Oskar Estebany, who had an intent to heal, held the mice in group one for fifteen minutes, twice a day. Medical students, who had no intent to heal, held the mice in group two, twice a day. The mice in the third group were a control, and received no treatment. After two weeks, researchers measured the wound sizes of each group of mice. The mice treated by Oskar Estebany had significantly smaller wounds. Statistical analysis demonstrated that the probability of this being a chance occurrence was less than one in one thousand.

In 1964, Dr. Grad studied the effects of treating "sick" barley seeds with the laying on of hands.[3] He soaked the seeds in a saline solution to make them sick, then divided them into three groups. The first group was watered with tap water, and the second group with water from flasks that had been held by persons disinterested in the experiment. The third group was watered from a flask held by Oskar Estebany for fifteen minutes each day. The barley seeds watered from Estebany's flask sprouted more seedlings, grew taller, and had more chlorophyll than the seeds watered from other flasks.

Dr. Krieger was aware of these studies, but she could find very little in the existing scientific and medical literature about the laying on of hands as applied to humans. She therefore designed her own research. To see if hands-on healing would cause any physiological changes in humans, Dr. Krieger studied its effects on the hemoglobin level in the blood. Hemoglobin is the oxygen-carrying molecule of red blood cells, and is analogous to plant chlorophyll. Because Dr. Grad's study on the barley seeds had demonstrated an increase in their chlorophyll level after being held by Colonel Estebany, Dr. Krieger postulated that the hemoglobin level in humans would increase after an individual was treated by laying on of hands.

To test her hypothesis, she first did a pilot study, then followed it by two other studies. In the pilot study, done in 1971, Dr. Krieger studied nineteen people who received laying on of hands by Oskar Estebany, and nine patients who received no treatment. The group members Estebany treated had an increase in their hemoglobin when researchers tested their blood four hours later. The control group—those untreated—did not.[4]

In 1972 Dr. Krieger replicated her study using a larger number of people. Oskar Estebany treated forty-three people. Thirty-three others served as controls and were not treated. The groups were comparable in sex and age. Once again, the treated group showed an increase in its members' hemoglobin levels four hours after being treated, while the control group did not.[5] In yet another study done in 1973, with approximately the same number of people, the results were the same. In this study, Dr. Krieger controlled for many other variables that might affect hemoglobin values, such as smoking, diet, medications, practice of meditation, breathing exercises by subjects who did yoga, and biorhythm change. The statistical analysis of these results demonstrated that the probability of the hemoglobin levels increasing by chance alone was less than one in one thousand.[6]

As a result of her research, Dr. Krieger concluded that the laying on of hands as practiced by an experienced healer had physiological effects. Meanwhile, Dora Kunz was developing a healing method, based on her earlier observations of healers, that she and Dolores Krieger could teach to nurses. They called this technique Therapeutic Touch, and began to teach it to Dr. Krieger's students. After a number of nurses had learned Therapeutic Touch, Dr. Krieger designed an experiment[7] to determine if the nurses could affect the patients' hemoglobin levels, just as Oskar Estebany had.

Dr. Krieger selected thirty-two nurses to participate in the study. Sixteen nurses treated two patients each with Therapeutic Touch, using a standardized technique that they had learned from either Dora Kunz or Dolores Krieger. Sixteen nurses provided regular nursing care, without using Therapeutic Touch. Before treatment, there was no significant difference in the mean hemoglobin of the groups, and the age distribution and gender makeup of each group were similar—all characteristics that affect hemoglobin level. Each nurse in the study treated two patients, for a total of sixty-four in the study. Technicians drew blood samples at comparable times for all participants. Researchers used the same machine to test all the blood samples, and the laboratory personnel were unaware that a study was under way. The group treated with

Therapeutic Touch had an increase in their hemoglobin level after treatment, but the group that received regular nursing care did not.

Dr. Krieger was one of the first to explore whether there was a scientific basis to results seen from healing with laying on of hands. Her studies provided a rationale for developing Therapeutic Touch as a tool for health professionals. She demonstrated that nurses trained in a standardized Therapeutic Touch technique could have similar physiological effects as Oskar Estebany, and supported Dora Kunz's hypothesis that the ability to heal could be taught. At the same time, nurses practicing Therapeutic Touch with their patients reported that it seemed to stimulate the body's natural healing processes. Because both research and clinical experience were promising, Dr. Krieger decided that she should teach Therapeutic Touch to health professionals. She developed a course proposal at the Division of Nursing at New York University to teach Therapeutic Touch at the master's level. The Dean's Advisory Committee approved the course, and formal instruction began in the fall of 1975. Since that time, Therapeutic Touch has expanded so that it is practiced extensively by thousands of health professionals throughout the United States, Canada, and Australia. These are mostly nurses, but an increasing number of physicians, psychotherapists, physical therapists, licensed massage therapists, and naturopathic physicians are integrating Therapeutic Touch techniques into their practices. From their work over the past twenty years, practitioners have compiled valuable information about the clinical effects of Therapeutic Touch, and have begun to investigate it scientifically. In the chapters that follow we will describe much of what practitioners and researchers have discovered about Therapeutic Touch and its ability to accelerate the body's healing.

The Human Energy Field

THERAPEUTIC TOUCH is based on the belief that the human being is a complex system of energy. While this is an ancient concept, it is a foreign one to most people living in Western societies. Western science and medicine tend to view an individual as having a physical body and a mind, which function because of a complex series of biochemical reactions. From this perspective, a human being lives by taking in food which through a series of chemical reactions releases energy.

Therapeutic Touch practitioners, while acknowledging this conventional view, also consider an individual to be a system of energy. They postulate the existence of physical, mental, emotional, and intuitive energies, which correspond to the unique characteristics of human beings. In health, our body, feelings, thoughts, and intuition work together to allow us to function in an integrated way.

The idea of the human being as a system of energy is supported by two diverse sources. One is Eastern philosophy, and the other is the contemporary nursing theory of Martha Rogers. From the perspective of some Eastern philosophies, the universe is composed of interacting systems of energy, derived from a unified source. In this worldview, there is an underlying unity to all consciousness, of which an individual is a localized expression. From the perspective of nursing educator Martha Rogers, the human being is a vibrating field of energy characterized by the ability to maintain its integrity, and to establish its own unique patterning. Rogers also conceptualizes each individual as an open system, continually exchanging information in the form of thoughts and feelings, both with other people and with the environment. She believes that healing involves a strengthening of the underlying integrity of an individual's human energies, and their repatterning in a healthier way.

At the time that Martha Rogers was developing her theories, both Dolores Krieger and Dora Kunz independently postulated the existence of human energies, and theorized that they could interact in a specific way to promote healing. Their view is similar to that of healers in many other cultures. Chinese, Indian, and Native American people, for example, share this belief in the individual as a system of energy that is in constant motion during life. In these systems of thought, one individual, acting as healer, can help another by assisting in the repatterning of their energy, and the reestablishment of its rhythmic flow.

Among other cultural healing practices, Chinese medicine is perhaps the best known in the West. At its foundation is a belief in the existence of *Qi* (or *ch'i*), a word used to describe the dynamic flow of life energy. *Qi* defies exact description in our language. It refers to a life force, or a vital force, that permeates living things, and departs when they die. *Qi* represents flow. It describes a life principle that is constantly changing, with a rhythm that is characteristic to each individual. From the Chinese perspective, *Qi* constantly circulates within the system. In health, there is balance and harmony within, and in relation to, the world outside. If this flow becomes disordered, illness may result.

The flow of *Qi* throughout the body is organized into path-

ways, called meridians. These pathways of flow are analogous to the circulatory system, which Western physiologists
have delineated. Just as the blood vessels of the body move
throughout the tissues carrying oxygen and nutrients, the meridians represent the organized flow of the vital energy, or
Qi. Along the meridians are various points, which the acu-
puncturist stimulates either with pressure or small needles.
This regulates the flow of *Qi*. Because each meridian has an
energetic link to a specific organ in the body, the acupuncture
practitioner improves the flow to vital organs of the body by
balancing the energy flow in the meridian. This promotes the
patient's overall health.

Just as Chinese culture believes in the vital principle of Qi,
Indian culture believes in a form of energy called prana. In-
dians consider prana to be an energizing life force, which is
available from the environment and flows throughout all living things. Prana represents a link among all life forms and
reinforces a unity that underlies the diversity of all life. In the
Indian worldview, pranic flow responds to an individual's
thoughts and emotions. Positive thoughts and emotions increase the amount of prana available to the body, which in
turn improves physical health. Maintaining psychological
health, therefore, becomes an important way to promote
physical health.

Many Native American cultures view the individual as a
system of energy comprised of physical, psychological, and
spiritual components. In health, these energies are in balance
with one another and there is a resonance that exists between
them. That is, the physical, psychological, and spiritual energies work together to support an individual who is integrated within, and is in harmony with the community.

Within the belief system of some Native Americans, each
organ of the body has a characteristic energy, with its own
rhythm. In a healthy person, each organ resonates with other

organs of the body. In a sick person, there may be a change in the rhythm of the diseased organ's energy, and a loss of the resonance between this organ and the other healthy parts of the body. The idea of the individual as a system of rhythmic energy is at the basis of the use of songs, chants, and drumming as a method for healing. Because music is composed of sound waves vibrating at a particular frequency and because it represents rhythm and order, Native American healing rituals often include its use to help restore the underlying harmony to the patient's energy.[1]

The ancient Greeks used music for healing, as well. The best known of these is Pythagoras, who lived during the sixth century B.C. Pythagoras believed that the individual was a collection of energies, and that illness represented a partial disharmony of the psychic nature. He believed in the healing power of sound, used to harmonize the patient's energy. He and his students used music to balance the energy flow of the sick person, and to assist the patient's energy to become a part of what Pythagoras felt was a universal process of flow and change. Pythagoras emphasized that sound was a way of communicating both the compassion of the healer and the intent of the healer that the patient be well.[2]

Although the idea that a nonmaterial energetic force is associated with living things has guided the healing practices of some other cultures, scientists have yet to characterize this force. However, modern physics has contributed to a greater understanding of the underlying characteristics of matter. There are three important concepts that suggest that living beings may be associated with nonmaterial energetic forces. The first of these is the existence of force fields. The second is the equivalence of matter and energy. The third is the discovery of the dynamic nature of the subatomic particles that are the structural basis of matter.

Force Fields

In the late seventeenth century, Sir Isaac Newton proved mathematically the laws of gravity. Since his contribution, scientists have known that large planetary bodies attract other bodies to themselves. The planets, the sun, and the moon have a gravitational field surrounding them, and they exert their attractive effects within the boundaries of that field. Although the field itself is not visible to the senses, its effects are measurable.

In the late nineteenth century, Michael Faraday and James Clerk Maxwell demonstrated the existence of electrical and magnetic fields. Through their work, they showed that electrical and magnetic fields, although nonmaterial themselves, could affect the behavior of matter. Iron filings, for example, when exposed to a magnet, will scatter in a way that demonstrates the boundaries of the magnet's field. When electromagnetic fields were first described, scientists believed them to be disturbances in empty space. Einstein, however, realized that electromagnetic fields were distinct entities that propagated through space, and that light itself was an electromagnetic field that travels in the form of waves.[3]

In addition to gravitational and electromagnetic fields, physicists have described nuclear force fields, which are wave fields associated with the elementary particles that comprise the atom.[4] These waves spread through space, and each wave contains a certain amount of energy.[5] Since atoms form molecules, and molecules eventually form organs and tissues, nuclear force fields are associated with living beings. Fritz Kunz, the mathematician and educator, wrote:

As years go by, more and more we are obliged to think of things as localizations of fields . . . The interrelation of the field and the appropriate objects is established at the microcosmic level, such as that of the atom. Since molecules, molar particles and great aggregates of substances are made up of atoms, the field is everywhere present in the object.[6]

Equivalence of Matter and Energy

We know from Albert Einstein's development of relativity theory that matter and energy are equivalent. The elementary particles composing the atom represent the smallest units of matter. When these particles collide with one another (as happens both experimentally, and in nature when they are exposed to cosmic radiation) the very high energy of the colliding particles transforms into mass. From this energy of motion, new particles form. The physicist Werner Heisenberg writes:

> The elementary particles of modern physics can be transformed into each other . . . They do not themselves consist of matter, but they are the only possible forms of matter. Energy becomes matter by taking on the form of an elementary particle, by manifesting itself in this form. [7]

The Dynamic Nature of Atomic Structure

In the early twentieth century, Niels Bohr, Albert Einstein, Werner Heisenberg, Louis de Broglie, Erwin Schrödinger, and others explored the structure and behavior of the atom. As a result of their work, we now have a model of the material world as one that is fundamentally dynamic.

The atom, a basic component of matter, consists of a nucleus, surrounded by a number of electrons. These electrons orbit at varying distances from the nucleus of the atom. The number of electrons in orbit may differ, depending on the substance. The original model of the atom was that of electrons orbiting the nucleus, in a fixed manner, as planets orbit the sun. That is, each electron had a specific place to circle the nucleus, and it always remained there.

In 1913, however, Niels Bohr postulated something different. He was aware that in 1900, Max Planck had investigated the radiation of energy from thermal bodies. Planck determined that the electrons responsible for radiation emission did so by emitting energy in bursts. These bursts were specific, discontinuous amounts of energy, which he called quanta.

Niels Bohr applied Planck's theory to a new model for the structure of the the atom. He suggested that the electron orbits the nucleus in a place that is characterized by a fixed amount of energy, but that it is not confined to this place. It may jump to a place of lesser energy, and when it does so, it emits a packet, or quanta, of energy. The electron may also jump to an orbit that is a further distance from the nucleus, and this requires that it absorb energy to do so. This jump of the electron is the so-called quantum leap. What is unusual about the quantum leap is that, according to Bohr, the observer cannot detect the electron passing through the space between orbits. It simply is at one level, or the other. It is as if the electron disappears in one place, and reappears in another.

Physicists are also aware that particles confined to small regions of space move at very high velocities. Within the structure of the atom, electrons are very confined and therefore are in constant motion. Fritjof Capra, a physicist with an interest in the philosophical implications of modern science, describes this characteristic motion:

> Inside the vibrating atoms, the electrons are bound to
> the atomic nuclei by electric forces that try to keep them

as close as possible, and they respond to this confinement by whirling around extremely fast. In the nuclei, finally, protons and neutrons are pressed into a minute volume by the strong nuclear forces, and consequently race about at unimaginable velocities.

Modern physics thus pictures matter not at all as passive and inert but as being in a continuous dancing and vibrating motion whose rhythmic patterns are determined by the molecular, atomic and nuclear configurations. [8]

Physicists have debated the philosophical significance of quantum mechanics since they first developed the theories, and they are not all in agreement. What is important here is that the model of the composition of matter has become different from what it was during the time of Newton. Matter is no longer considered inert. The basic components of matter are particles that are constantly emitting and absorbing energy, changing position, yet at the same time maintaining equilibrium. There is an underlying dynamism associated with material objects, although it may not always be visible to the naked eye. At the basis of life are subatomic particles, continually in motion and continually emitting or taking in energy. Living beings, by virtue of their molecular makeup, participate in this energy.

A Theory of Human Energy Fields

In the early 1980s, Dora Kunz and others developed a theory of human energy fields that serves as a model for understanding human interaction. Their ideas also help us to understand the basis of disease, and the way to promote health. From their perspective, each person is a localization of energy—a kind of force field. This individual energy field exists in a larger sea of energy, a universal energy field, from which it draws energy, and to which it gives energy. This implies that all living things are interconnected. But, although each person shares in this universal energy, he also has a separate identity. He has a focus of awareness that he experiences as himself.

This theory was developed from the ideas of Fritz Kunz, who, as mentioned earlier, hypothesized that living things are localizations of force fields. He emphasized that:

—Empty space is not empty, but at any point in the universe there are force field potentials.
—These fields obey predictable laws, and provide a stable background for the events of our world.
—Fields interact, and fields exchange energy.
—Every living thing occurs within a force field, and in fact can be thought of as a localization of the field. [9]

Although scientists have no clear understanding of the exact nature of the force field that characterizes living beings, the model proposed by Dora Kunz and others describes the human energy field as consisting of properties unique to human beings. In a series of papers, *Fields and their Clinical Implications*, Dora Kunz and Dr. Erik Peper describe an individual as made up of physical, emotional, mental, and intuitive energies.[10]

Therapeutic Touch is based on this idea that the human being is a system of energy. The human energy field has several components that work together to maintain health.

The Physical Field

There is a characteristic energy, which Therapeutic Touch practitioners call physical energy, that is specifically associated with the physical body. All living creatures have physical energy, which flows through the body and energizes our organs and tissues. In a healthy person there is a surplus of physical energy.

While physical energy is flowing through the body, it moves with a characteristic rhythm. The energy associated with each organ of the body has a *specific* rhythm, and in health there is a free transfer of energy between the organs of the body. Illness or surgery disrupts this harmonious flow. If an organ is diseased or removed, this disturbs the usual rhythm, and as part of the healing process, the physical energy must reorganize itself.

During Therapeutic Touch, a trained practitioner uses her hands to detect disruption to the physical energy flow, and helps the energy to move freely again. In ways we will describe in more detail in Chapter Three, this promotes the body's natural healing process.

The Emotional Field

The emotional field contains the energy associated with feeling. This includes positive feeling, such as happiness, concern for others, and joy, as well as the more painful emotions of anger, fear, and resentment. The emotional energy surrounds and interpenetrates the physical energy. Emotions, therefore, have a profound effect on how the body functions.

Because our emotions naturally go outward, they can affect others. We all are, to some extent, sensitive to what other people feel. For example, many of us have experienced a feeling of peace when in the presence of someone who is relaxed and calm. We are even more sensitive to the emotion of another if he directs it *specifically* toward us. If we are with a friend who is angry at us, for example, we feel this more intensely than if we are in the presence of a person who is angry, but not directly at us. Through this experience of shared emotion, we feel connection with others. In this way our emotions are part of a shared universal emotional field.

Every time we feel something, we set our energy in motion. This affects the overall flow and rhythm of our energy, especially if we are feeling the same way repeatedly. Persistent positive emotions enhance our energy flow, but negative emotions that are constant and repetitive can disrupt the flow, or slow it down. Because the emotional and physical energy are connected, disruptions in the emotional energy can, over time, affect the amount of energy available to the body, and in this way affect physical health.

During Therapeutic Touch, the practitioner takes advantage of her emotional connection to the patient. She becomes calm, which sets up a rhythm in her own emotional field, and projects this feeling toward the patient. Almost always the patient will begin to feel peaceful and to relax. As we shall see in Chapter Five, the relaxation response plays an important physiological role in the healing process. Relaxation also allows the patient's energy to flow harmoniously, and increases the amount of energy available to the body for healing.

The Mental Field

The mental field represents our ability to think. Clear thinking is part of ourselves. In our daily lives we use rational thought to direct our activities and plan for the future; we also use our ability to think in order to understand and influence our emotions. In a different way, we use our ability to think in order to understand concepts and to be creative. This form of thought is more abstract, and is related to our use of intuition, which stimulates creative insight.

The mental energy of thought is associated with our emotional and physical energy. This means that there is a relationship between our thoughts and our feelings, as well as a connection between what we are thinking and feeling, and our physical health. Positive habitual patterns of thought and feeling stimulate the flow of energy available to the physical body. This promotes health. Persistent negative patterns of thought and feeling partially inhibit the amount of energy available to the body. This lowering of the body's energy may put us at higher risk for illness.

The ability to think clearly is something that human beings all share. That is, there is a shared mental field that allows us to influence one another with our thoughts—our individual thoughts can reach outward toward others. Dora Kunz and Erik Peper explain this:

> . . . the mental field has the ability to radiate out a very small portion of itself over long distances, when directed by one's thoughts. For this field to reach out to others, it needs the impulse of a strong emotion such as love or anxiety. This . . . allows the mental field to reach out and resonate with the mental field of another person. [11]

During Therapeutic Touch, the practitioner makes a clear mental image of the patient as healthy. Because of their shared mental field, the practitioner's image can affect the recipient by helping to restore the body's order. The idea that the practitioner's thoughts affect the patient is not simply theoretical. As we will discuss in Chapter Three, research demonstrates that one person's mental images may affect the physiology of another who is nearby.

The Intuitional Field

Besides the body, emotions, and mind, Kunz and Peper describe intuition as a unique human characteristic. Intuition is a level of awareness that goes beyond rational thought, and is responsible for insight. Insight allows us to directly understand the truth of an idea all at once, without having to think it through logically. Intuition and insight underlies our ability to create.

The intuition of each of us joins us to a larger intuitional field, shared with all humans. This shared intuitional field gives each of us a feeling, even if only briefly, of connection to nature or another person.

Our physical health, feelings, and thoughts affect our ability to be aware of our intuition. When our mind and emotions are quiet and working in harmony with one another, and when our body relaxes, we are more responsive to intuition. Recipients of Therapeutic Touch frequently report that the mental and emotional calming induced by the treatment allows them to be more aware of their intuition. Recipients often describe, for example, that they have new insights into solving difficult personal problems, or gain new perspectives on their relationships.

The Dynamic Nature of Human Energy

Because our energy continually flows, we are always changing. Our experience with our bodies confirms this. The physical body renews and regenerates itself constantly. Bones and muscles remodel themselves, depending on external stresses. The organs of the body replace their cells in an orderly fashion. In the same way, our feelings change from moment to moment, and our thoughts may change rapidly as well.

All of our energies naturally intermingle. In health there is an integrated working together of our body, emotions, mind, and intuition. In illness there is disruption of this harmonious interaction. Because the body, mind, and emotions are not working together there is a decrease in the amount of energy available to the individual.

A healthy person openly exchanges energy with the world around. As we share experiences with others, we exchange ideas and feelings. Ideas and feelings are forms of energy that connect us to others through a medium of energy exchange, even if we are not speaking.

Because of this exchange, our feelings and thoughts can and do affect others, even though we may be unaware of it. As will become more apparent in later chapters, it is this energy exchange between people that provides a basis for Therapeutic Touch. During Therapeutic Touch, the practitioner helps to increase the energy in the patient's system. She also helps it to flow more rhythmically. The patient can then use this energy to promote the body's natural healing process.

3

Ideas About Healing

IN EVALUATING ANY form of healing, whether conventional medicine or unconventional therapies, we make basic assumptions about the healing process. Modern medicine has made great strides in understanding the mechanisms of disease, and in developing cures for many illnesses. Despite this, no one knows exactly how healing takes place. Although physicians understand some of the mechanics of healing—the role of the immune system in fighting infections, for example, and the biochemical step in wound repair—they remain unaware of all the ordering forces that guide the body in its maintenance of homeostasis. Even though scientists have recently become aware of the sophisticated communication between the brain and the body, they are far from understanding the complex intelligence, intrinsic to the human being, that maintains the orderly functioning of the whole.

Although a complete understanding of the healing process may be elusive, it is nevertheless important to examine our beliefs about healing, and as far as it is possible, to construct a model for how we think healing occurs. We act on the basis of our beliefs, whether we are patients or health care providers. Our ideas about healing will guide us in the kind of care we seek. If we are practitioners, they will guide us in the kind of care we give.

Therapeutic Touch is based on three fundamental beliefs. First, there is a universal healing energy, available to all, that has order as its basis. Second, there is an underlying unity among life forms: Our interconnectedness allows one person to help another. Third, what we think and how we feel can affect our physical health. A sick person, therefore, plays an active role in the healing process.

Order as a Basis for Healing

Order is an underlying characteristic of the universe. This statement may seem unusual on the face of it, because we live in a rapidly changing world, which often seems chaotic. While it is true that change is a feature of life, there is also an underlying organization to our experience. As mentioned in Chapter Two, both gravitational and electromagnetic fields provide a stable, consistent background for material existence, and illustrate an ordering principle. They establish certain conditions that we take for granted in our daily lives. For example, the laws of planetary motion do not change. We expect the earth to remain in orbit around the sun, and that the moon will exert predictable effects on the tides. In the same way, the consistency of the behavior of electrical fields allows us to generate electrical current, deliver it to our homes and offices, and use it reliably to turn on lights, television sets, and computers.

Order is also a characteristic of living systems. Although living things experience change—our bodies change on a day-to-day basis, and our emotions may change from moment to moment—there is an organizing principle that allows us to function as coherent wholes. This ability to be self-organizing is a fundamental property of living systems. The human body is an obvious example of this. The bodies of complex living creatures have many specialized tissues that group together to form organs. All of these organs have specific functions, and they work together to maintain the integrity of the whole. If illness damages one organ of the body, others may partially compensate for its function, in order to preserve the overall ability of the whole to work together.

The physiological response that occurs with blood loss is an excellent example of this. If a person experiences the sudden loss of a large amount of blood, the body, through the action of hormones secreted by the sympathetic nervous system and adrenals, will immediately begin to readjust its blood flow. The circulation to the hands, feet, and large skeletal muscles will slow down, in order to preserve the flow of blood to the brain, heart, and kidneys. At the same time, the heart will beat more times per minute to compensate for the fact that it is sending less blood per beat to the body. The kidneys respond by releasing ADH, a hormone that allows the body to conserve water. They also secrete renin, a substance that promotes sodium retention and helps maintain blood pressure. Through this complex series of events the organs work together to compensate for the blood loss, and help the body maintain homeostasis.

In a more complex way, the body, emotions, and mind of a person also interact in an orderly manner. In a healthy person, they are integrated and contribute to a sense of well-being, and an ability to make a contribution to others. A carpenter who builds a house, for example, needs a healthy body that can perform the physical task. He also needs a mental concept of how to build the house, and the emotional stability and strength of will to continue to work on the project, despite any setbacks he encounters. An airplane pilot needs the physical coordination to fly a plane, but also needs to understand what he is doing, and needs the emotional control to function effectively in an emergency. In these and other everyday situations, it is the body, mind, and emotions *working together* that permits successful completion of most human tasks.

If we think of health not as simply the absence of disease, but as the ability to participate fully in life, then to be healthy requires this integrated functioning of the body, emotions, and mind. Health also implies we have capacity to be creative. When we are sick, however, instead of integration, order, and creativity, there is some degree of disorder. When viewed from this perspective, healing involves the restoration of order, and the promotion of greater integration within the sick person.

Modern science has made great headway in understanding how the body, mind, and emotions interrelate. Scientists know that the brain and the body communicate with one another by means of transmitters called peptides. These peptides, which are amino acids strung together, shuttle between the brain and the body. They allow the brain to send messages to the autonomic nervous system, which regulates our response to stress. They also allow the brain to communicate with the immune system, which protects the body against infections and cancer. Neuropeptides, in addition, allow the brain to direct the functioning of the endocrine system, which is responsible for our hormonal balance.

The body communicates with the brain, as well, by sending messages from the immune, endocrine, and autonomic nervous system. Because of this two-way communication, some of which is almost instantaneous, we can conceptualize the body and mind as working together in an integrated way. Scientists also understand that emotional states have a major effect on the functioning of the body and mind. There are areas in the brain that are associated with emotion, and that both receive and send information in the form of peptides. These molecules communicate with other areas in the brain, and with the body as well. The limbic system, which processes emotion, has neural connections with the frontal lobes, which play an important role in conscious thought. Both these areas are connected to the hypothalamus, which plays a key role in regulating the autonomic nervous system, the hormonal balance of the body, and the immune system. [1]

Despite the gains of science in understanding the means of body-mind communication, there is as yet no all-encompassing theory that explains the ability of living creatures to maintain their complex order. However, some scientists have tried to explain the tendency of living things to be self-organizing. Biologists have noted that as living forms develop, their structure becomes more complex. For example, a human begins life as an embryo that initially contains two cells. From this simple structure, a complex organism develops, with specialized tissues and organs. What explains the ability of the embryo to direct its own development?

The British biologist Rupert Sheldrake has theorized that there exists what he calls morphogenetic fields, which guide the orderly development of living things. He suggests that morphogenetic fields are similar to gravitational and electromagnetic fields. Although all are invisible, they are real. We know them, not through our senses, but through their effects. He describes morphogenetic fields as nonmaterial spatial patterns—a type of abstract blueprint—which control the development of living forms.[2]

He postulates that the development of living systems is guided both by DNA, and what he calls "something more than DNA." The something more is the morphogenetic field that contains and transmits the overall pattern that the developing form will take. He suggests that the existence of morphogenetic fields explains "how cells group together in tissues of particular forms; and how those are shaped into organisms of particular forms."[3]

Sheldrake's ideas, somewhat controversial among his peers, are interesting because they suggest that a nonmaterial pattern directs the ordering of form. In this way, Sheldrake's theory resembles the ideas of Plato. Plato believed that material objects—living and inanimate—pattern themselves after abstract form. These forms are archetypes, or perfect models for the material object. Plato considers the forms to be permanent and unchanging, unlike the objects of our material reality, which he considers imperfect and transient copies of the abstract forms. Dr. Renee Weber, a Philosophy professor at Rutgers University, has written on the philosophical foundation of healing. She suggests that Platonic philosophy contains a model for healing. In describing Plato's theory she writes:

> ... the ... nature of any given entity depends upon its correctly reproducing the eternal, essential Platonic form in whose "image" it is made. In the case of living organisms, for example, proper "participation" in the Form translates into health, whereas faulty participation leads to illness ... [4]

From the Platonic point of view, then, optimal health depends on how well the form and function of a person aligns with an abstract image of his perfection.

In addition to Sheldrake and Plato, the physicist David Bohm suggests that there is a nonmaterial ordering basis to our experience. He calls this the implicate order, in which all things exist as a unified whole. He theorizes that it provides a background for our everyday world of material objects, which he calls the explicate order.[5]

All three of these thinkers—Sheldrake, Bohm, and Plato—believe that there is an abstract pattern at work to explain the order we experience in our usual world. The theories they espouse suggest that our material reality derives from a nonmaterial reality. If we apply this idea to healing, it implies that the more subtle energy, such as that of thought and emotion, has an effect on our physical health. Although at present it is impossible for science to verify whether or not there exist abstract patterns for order, we do know that our thoughts and emotions affect the physical functioning of the body. A specific example of this is the well-accepted technique of biofeedback, which demonstrates that what we think has an effect on our physiological processes.

Through biofeedback, a patient learns to voluntarily control physical functions such as heart rate, muscle tension, and blood pressure and blood flow to some parts of his body. He receives feedback from an instrument that monitors the function he is controlling: Usually a light or a tone emitted by the machine tells the patient when he is successful. The patient controls his body not by actively trying, but by directed thinking, which includes mental imagery. If the patient imagines lifting a heavy object, for example, the biofeedback apparatus will record an increase in electrical activity in the muscle. This indicates that the muscle is contracting.

Health care practitioners have used biofeedback successfully to treat common medical problems. These include cardiac arrhythmia, migraine headache, circulatory problems such as Raynaud's disease, and chronic pain. The success of biofeedback depends to some extent on the skill of the practitioner who instructs the patient. However, psychophysiologist Jeanne Achterberg believes that it is the subject's ability to use his imagination that plays the major role in determining the effectiveness of biofeedback. In a study that examined the success of biofeedback in training patients with rheumatoid arthritis to relax, she noted that the patients with the best response were those who were most successful at imagining their own health.[6] The patients who had difficulty learning biofeedback were those who could not fantasize.

With biofeedback, a patient, through the power of

thought, is able to have some effect on his own body. With Therapeutic Touch, the practitioner uses thought to imagine another person as well. There is some experimental basis for the belief that the practitioner's mental image may affect the patient's physiology and the way he feels. In 1983, William Braud and Marilyn Schlitz, at the Mind Science Foundation in San Antonio, Texas, studied the effect of mental images, sent at a distance to thirty-two subjects.[7] The researchers designed the study to determine if people designated as influencers could affect the sympathetic nervous system activity of the subjects. Specifically, the influencers attempted to calm the subjects, by sending them calming mental images or feelings of quiet. The subjects were in a separate room, twenty meters away from the influencers. To determine if the influencers had any effect on the subjects, the researchers measured the change in electrical current conducted through the subjects' skin. (The conduction of current through the skin, its electrodermal activity, is a measure of the electrical activity of the sweat glands, which are innervated by fibers from the sympathetic nervous system. High electrodermal activity is consistent with stress or arousal; low activity is consistent with a state of calm.)

At the start of the study, researchers identified sixteen of the subjects as having higher sympathetic nervous system arousal, and therefore being in greater need of calming. The other sixteen were designated as *calm* and were not in particular need of further calming. The researchers discovered that the influencers were able to calm the more aroused subjects to a significant extent, but did not have the same effect on the subjects who were already calm.

The results of this study suggest that it is possible for one person, through the use of mental images, and by a focused intent, to affect the physiology of another person nearby. Of note, as well, is that the influencers had the most success with the subjects who had the greatest need for calming—the ones with the high sympathetic nervous system activity. The researchers hypothesized that the need for calming had made the subjects somehow more receptive to help.

From the Therapeutic Touch practitioner's perspective, the results of this study are not surprising if we think of a human being as a system that is in open communication with the environment. In Chapter Two, we considered the existence of thought as a radiating pattern of energy that affects not only the thinker, but others in the vicinity. If we hypothesize that our thoughts extend out over a distance, then it is possible for the practitioner's thought to affect a patient who is nearby. In fact, clinical experience demonstrates that when the practitioner imagines the patient as healthy and calm during a Therapeutic Touch treatment, the patient almost always relaxes. Like the subjects of the study by Braud and Schlitz, the patient receiving Therapeutic Touch responds somewhat to the internal state of the practitioner. Because the patient does respond to the thoughts and feelings of others, and because Therapeutic Touch practitioners believe that order is a basis for healing, they always think of order being restored within the body when they treat their patients. At present, it is impossible to prove scientifically that the practitioner's thought of order is what actually promotes the healing process. As we will discuss in Chapter Five, however, the effects of Therapeutic Touch which have been studied so far suggest that both the practitioner's projection of calm and the focused idea of restoring order contribute to an acceleration of healing.

Integration and Unity

The practice of Therapeutic Touch rests on the belief that there is an underlying unity that all life forms share. From this point of view, healing implies not only that order is restored within the individual, but also that balance and harmony are restored in the sick person's relationships with others. Healing suggests, in addition, that the sick person returns to a contributing role in society.

These ideas reflect the fact that none of us lives in isolation, but are part of a larger, unified web of relationships. This perspective on healing is an integrative one. It differs, to some extent, from the beliefs that are implicit in the practice of conventional Western medicine. Although modern medical practice has much to offer, it is fundamentally mechanistic and fragmented in its approach.

Many physicians recognize that their patients have an innate recuperative power. They also know that the body has a drive to maintain its order. Most physicians are now aware that thoughts and feelings play some role in the physical health of their patients. Despite these insights, practitioners often deliver medical care in a fragmented way. Doctors sometimes approach illness predominantly as a malfunction of a body part or as a biochemical abnormality, which they can correct by choosing the appropriate drug. Illness is also reduced to mechanical failure, which can be repaired by surgery. While at times these approaches may be therapeutic, they are incomplete if practitioners ignore the mental, emotional, and social contributors to illness.

In our modern era of specialization, the patient runs the risk of being referred to a different specialist for each part of the body, but never being considered as a whole human being. Certainly specialization in science and medicine is often an appropriate way of focusing on a defined area to understand it more fully. However, if the specialist focuses only on one aspect of the patient, while ignoring the context of the whole, his care may become fragmented. Even when the patient receives appropriate scientific care, he often feels something is missing.

The risk of fragmentation is an outgrowth of the scientific

approach. To study something scientifically requires that the thinker separate himself from the object. The thinker becomes a spectator, building a body of logical knowledge about something that he considers to be an impersonal *it*. The scientific approach is inherently dualistic—the thinking self is always separate from, or outside, what is under consideration.

Modern scientific thinking derives from the seventeenth-century contributions of René Descartes, who, besides being a philosopher, was a mathematician. Descartes believed that problems should be approached analytically—that they should be broken into parts and ordered logically. His method was reductionistic: He believed that we could unravel complex problems by understanding the components.

Besides Descartes, Galileo also had a major effect on modern science. In about 1600, he postulated that scientists should restrict themselves to studying those things that they could measure. This represented a shift away from the earlier role of science, which was predominantly that of classification. When science embraced measurement, it turned away from consideration of anything that was not verifiable in this way. Ken Wilber comments on this in his book *The Spectrum of Consciousness*. He writes:

> . . . assurance of human happiness was promised by the new science of measurement . . . Ultimate Reality was that which could be measured . . . All propositions were to be confined to that which was objectively measurable . . . (If) something didn't submit to these criteria, then it just did not exist or plainly was not worth knowing.[8]

It is important to keep in mind that the Scientific Revolution, with its emphasis on analytic thinking and measurement, represented a great leap forward for humanity. Prior to this time, the Church was the primary authority in matters scientific. Science was based not only on reason, but also on acceptance of some ideas as a matter of faith. The Middle Ages, in addition, were a time when people interpreted events solely based on their own personal, cultural, and religious experiences.[9] The introduction of analysis and measurement allowed humankind to step away from an immersion in its own experience and to look more objectively at the world and its workings.

As a result of our ability to reason and to measure, and to separate ourselves from the objects that we study, we have developed a sophisticated technology that benefits us all. Medical applications of technology, for example, have provided us with sophisticated diagnostic techniques such as magnetic resonance imaging, which allows highly accurate pictures to be taken of many parts of the body. This represents a use of technology that has spared sick people painful medical procedures that used to be necessary to arrive at medical diagnoses.

However, with Western culture so heavily influenced by the reductionism of scientific thinking, something has been lost. Before the Scientific Revolution, and the Industrial Revolution that it spawned, the average person lived in a closer relationship with nature. Most individuals worked on the land and understood in a more personal sense that it was the means of their survival. People were dependent on one another because communities were smaller and more isolated. Each person often had a specific skill, and filled a unique role. People experienced a sense of interdependence and of being a contributing part of the whole.

With the advent of reductionistic thinking in the 1600s, and the Industrial Revolution that followed, the machine became the metaphor for our existence. This metaphor was applied to the physical world, and living things as well. From the perspective of scientific medicine, the human being became analogous to a machine that physicians could repair by attending to its malfunctioning parts. Although this way of looking at the world has enriched our understanding of our makeup, it can also lead to an emphasis on the functioning of the parts, at the expense of considering the integrated, unified whole.

The psychologist Charles Johnston believes that Western culture, by overemphasizing the mechanistic and rational approach to understanding, has sacrificed participation in the flow of the dynamic, creative process of life. In describing this he writes:

> . . . what is missing is life. In Newtonian/Cartesian reality the universe and all within it are like a great clockworks, an immense and wondrous machinery. A mechanical paradigm can offer us many amazing things. But no matter how great a machine's complexity, it can never be more than just that, a machine.[10]

We think of healing as a way of assisting a person to participate more fully in the creative process of life. Healing implies that the sick person not only becomes free of physical symptoms, but also that the body, mind, emotions, and creativity of the patient work together more effectively. Therapeutic Touch is successful as an adjunct to medical care because it promotes healing in a way that emphasizes this underlying wholeness of the patient. Although patients receiving Therapeutic Touch may or may not experience some improvement of their physical condition, most report feeling more at peace and less anxious about their illness. Some patients also say that their relationships with family members have improved, or that they have had a creative insight about how to solve a serious problem in their lives.

Janice, a woman in her thirties, sought Therapeutic Touch to help her high blood pressure. She hoped that Therapeutic Touch would do away with the need for medication to control her blood pressure. The practitioner explained that although Therapeutic Touch might be helpful, it was impossible to guarantee that she would no longer need medication. Janice wished to try Therapeutic Touch in hope of some improvement, but agreed to continue to see her physician for treatment of her blood pressure. After four treatments, Janice's blood pressure improved to the extent that her doctor discontinued one of her medications. But, even more important, she began to realize that her job was placing her under great stress. As a studious and quiet person, she had enjoyed her job as a librarian at a university. When the director of the library appointed her to supervise other librarians, she found her job stressful. She was constantly embroiled in staff disputes, or solving personnel problems. The occupation she had loved was now making her unhappy.

After a series of Therapeutic Touch treatments, Janice decided to make plans for another career in computer science. She realized that she was not suited for working with large numbers of people, and wanted a job more compatible with her introverted personality. She was relieved and optimistic after making her decision.

It is possible, of course, that a patient's decision to change her life was merely coincidental with her Therapeutic Touch treatments. Based on the clinical experience with Therapeutic Touch over the past twenty years, however, it is a relatively common occurrence for patients to make life changes that bring their outer experience closer to who they feel they are inside. For Janice, getting better did not mean that her high blood pressure disappeared completely. Instead, she took more control over her life in order to eliminate the stress that was contributing to her hypertension.

Janice's experience with high blood pressure suggests that healing does not necessarily include a return of physical function. In fact, Janice experienced greater integration in her life, but only partial improvement physically. This stands in contrast to the mechanical model of healing, which too often narrowly defines health as return to physical function. Although the individual practitioner may have a broader view, conventional medical practice often operates *as if* return of function were the only goal of the healer.

Most physicians and nurses trained in Western countries have learned to equate healing with return of function of the ailing organ or body part. If we treat a patient's pneumonia with antibiotics and he recovers, he is restored to full function. If we treat a young adult's Hodgkin's disease (a kind of lymphatic cancer) with radiation and chemotherapy, he can fully recover. However, there are many patients who, despite the best of medical therapy, will never return to full function. Some cancer patients will eventually die from their disease. Many patients with autoimmune diseases, such as lupus or rheumatoid arthritis, will be helped to remission, but will experience recurrences of their illness. Most patients who are HIV infected will become sicker and eventually die despite the best of care. If nurses and physicians equate healing with return of function in the care of their patients, they are likely to feel frustrated and doomed to fail eventually, no matter what they do to help. But, if health care practitioners have a broader concept of healing as integration, they can assist their patients to live fully, despite their illness.

The Patient's Role in Healing

The patient plays an active role in the healing process. With Therapeutic Touch, as with any other healing interaction, some patients may respond more to treatment than others. Although it is not entirely clear why this is true, one factor that affects the response of the patient is his mental and emotional state.

Some patients are psychologically more receptive to Therapeutic Touch because they have less rigid emotional and mental patterns. If their beliefs about themselves are inflexible—if they believe that they cannot get better, for example—they may be less willing to accept help. This attitude can interfere with the patient's ability to relax during treatment. Relaxation allows the patient to take in more healing energy, while tension partially inhibits his ability to do so.

The way that a sick person thinks and feels about himself can affect the healing process in other ways, as well. If he thinks of himself as identified with the illness, it is more difficult to become well, because his self-image is that of a sick person. It is more helpful for the patient to acknowledge the illness, but not to identify with it. He can say to himself, "I have a disease," but at the same time realize that he is more than his illness. He can become aware that there is an inner "I," a self-awareness that persists, whether we are sick or well, and no matter what we are thinking or feeling. If the patient realizes that there is a part of himself that is whole, and unaffected by the illness, he can identify with this healthy inner self.

Friends, relatives, and caretakers of a sick person can help to enhance his self-image by encouraging the patient to reach out to others, and to become involved in creative activities. This increases his sense of health and vitality, and allows him to see that he can make a contribution, even if it is a small one. Patients who go outward to others reinforce for themselves the idea that they have the strength to participate in life and the strength to get better.

A patient who receives a diagnosis of a serious illness immediately begins to make mental pictures about what experiences await him in the future. These images may be of the pain and suffering he fears his illness will cause. Jonathan, newly diagnosed with HIV, the virus that causes AIDS, repeatedly envisioned wasting away and dying in pain, even though he felt well at the time of his diagnosis. Steven, when told he had cancer, began to fear repeated hospitalizations and saw himself in pain as a result of his cancer therapies. Although it is natural to worry about what the future will hold, both Jonathan and Steven, like many patients, risk becoming identified with their fearful pictures. They can become unable to separate their self-identity from the fearful images invoked by the diagnosis of illness. The mental pictures will often hover just outside their awareness, but come to the forefront when they are tired or in discomfort. This causes anxiety, and the patient feels emotionally drained. The patient's physicians, nurses, and family need to be aware that, at times, well-meaning comments about the illness can evoke fearful images for the sick person. Sometimes the mention of the diagnosis alone invokes an identification with the disease. Physicians, to whom the patient may attribute great power over the illness, should recognize that realistically hopeful comments may have a profoundly positive effect over how the patient sees himself and his possibility for improvement.

As Jeanne Achterberg points out in her book, *Imagery in Healing*, the body translates images into physical change. She describes images as a bridge between our conscious thoughts and our physiological functioning.[11] The cells of our immune system, for example, react to messages from the brain, mediated by our thoughts and images. Studies have shown that the patient's mental images have a direct effect on the functioning of the immune system. Drs. Barry L. Gruber and Nicholas Hall, in one study, demonstrated that cancer patients who used relaxation techniques, as well as their creative imagination, could stimulate lymphocyte production and enhance the activity of their natural killer (NK) cells. Both lymphocytes and NK cells play an active role in the body's destruction of cancer cells.[12]

Therapeutic Touch has a role in helping the patient to be less affected by his frightening images of pain and debilitation. Because the most powerful effect of Therapeutic Touch is relaxation, during the treatment the patient is usually free of anxiety. This helps the patient to learn that despite his illness, it is possible to be free from pain or anxiety and frightening mental pictures. The patient can return to the memory of the Therapeutic Touch treatment when his thoughts distress him, or he is in pain. In a more concrete way, he can associate his Therapeutic Touch treatment with a specific image that represents healing for him. Each year, several patients attend Therapeutic Touch workshops for health professionals on Orcas Island in the Pacific Northwest. During Therapeutic Touch treatments, which often take place outdoors, natural beauty surrounds the workshop participants. The patients often think of images from nature, such as a tree, as a symbol of peace, or a pain-free time. Many of the patients describe returning to these images for relief over the ensuing months, when they suffer from pain or anxiety.

For most people, healing occurs as a gradual process, where the physical illness improves, and the sick person slowly feels more vitality and integration. And in many cases, a patient may improve only partially. A person with cancer, for example, may experience remission, but later relapse, or a patient suffering from arthritis may have partial improvement of his pain. Cases of rapid and dramatic cure of illness are extremely rare, and we should not expect it from Therapeutic Touch, or any other medical or healing intervention.

Sudden and spontaneous remissions from disease have occurred, however, and researchers have analyzed some of these. Sudden cures appear related more to beliefs and attitudes of the patients than to their therapies. This is not to suggest that our beliefs and attitudes *alone* dictate whether or not we recover physically from serious illness. The causes of illness are often multifactorial and complex, and we are far from completely understanding why some people get better and some don't. However, when Elmer and Alyce Green studied four hundred cases of spontaneous remission, they discovered that the only common factor in these cases was the presence of hope for the future and a positive attitude toward life.[13] When Larry Dossey, in his book *Healing Words*,[14] reported on five cases of spontaneous regression documented at Kyushu University's School of Medicine in Japan, he listed some common characteristics of the patients. Among other things, they had an acceptance of their illness, an absence of anxiety and depression, and a continued interest in their activities. They made attempts to change aspects of their personality that led to difficulty in their relationships with others. The characteristics of the Japanese patients suggest that a positive attitude, a feeling that they were not powerless, and the ability to be flexible and adapt to their circumstances have some effect on the healing process.

Therapeutic Touch plays a role in helping a patient adapt to serious illness. Because it increases his energy, Therapeutic Touch often helps the sick person to cope with the stresses of illness in a more positive way. He may have more energy to participate in decisions about his care, which gives him a measure of control over his illness. He usually has more energy to participate in activities he finds rewarding, which supports his hopes for the future. The degree to which Therapeutic Touch is helpful to a patient depends, to some extent, on his underlying personality traits. Some people, for example, are more positive by nature and less threatened by the prospect of illness than others. Despite these differences, many people who receive Therapeutic Touch find it easier to identify with an inner self that remains unaffected by their illness, and therefore can continue to participate in life, despite the partial limitation of their disease.

Although we do not know exactly how healing occurs, it seems to be facilitated by the dynamic interaction where three factors play a role: the existence of a universal life energy with order as its basis, the intent of one person to help another, and the state of mind of the sick person, which affects his receptivity toward healing. Each of these factors makes its own contributions to the healing process. In ways that we will discuss more specifically in the next chapter, Therapeutic Touch practitioners can influence two of these factors: Through their clear intent to help another, they make a universal energy that restores order more available to the Therapeutic Touch recipient. The receptivity of the patient plays its own role in determining the effectiveness of healing.

4

The Method

ALL THERAPEUTIC TOUCH practitioners follow a specific method as they treat their patients.* One nurse describes what she does and how she feels while giving a Therapeutic Touch treatment:

> As I begin, I quiet my mind and consciously direct my attention within. Although I am aware of my surroundings, I ignore any distractions. I calm my emotions so that I feel peaceful and relaxed. In this frame of mind, I start to assess my patient: I pass my hands from head to foot a few inches over the surface of her body, while she sits in a chair, fully dressed. As I do this, my hands feel the subtle sensations that provide information about the flow of en-

---

*This chapter provides a brief description of the method of Therapeutic Touch. The reader who desires more detailed information is directed to Dolores Krieger's book, *The Therapeutic Touch*, and to *Therapeutic Touch, A Practical Guide*, by Janet Macrae. Although books are helpful, the best way to learn Therapeutic Touch is to take a workshop from an experienced practitioner, and to continue practicing. Like any other practical skill, it is best learned by doing.

ergy through the patient's body. I perceive this energy as a very light flowing sensation under my hands. As I assess each area of the body, I record mentally my impressions, and continue with the assessment.

At the end of the assessment I have information about the pattern of energy flow throughout the body, and I then begin to balance this flow of energy. Keeping my mind and emotions quiet, I project a feeling of peace toward the patient. At the same time, I move my hands rhythmically in a downward direction, six inches over the surface of the patient's body. I continue until I feel a smooth, even flow of energy under my hands. After a few minutes, I notice that the patient relaxes deeply.

When the patient's energy is balanced, I begin to direct energy to her. I don't draw on my own energy, but I think of myself as a conduit for a healing energy that passes through me, to the recipient. While I direct energy, I continue to keep my mind and emotions quiet. I make a mental image of the recipient as whole and well. I think of her body's order being restored, while I continue to project feelings of peace.

When I have finished directing energy to the patient, I rebalance its flow. When I can no longer detect any changes in the recipient's energy flow, I know that the treatment is coming to an end.

Whenever I treat with Therapeutic Touch, I feel connected to the patient. I feel both compassion and empathy. I always feel relaxed during the treatment, and my sense of time changes. Its passage seems to be suspended, even though I remain aware of a linear flow of events. When I treat with Therapeutic Touch, my thought process changes. My thinking becomes less cognitive and more intuitive—I sometimes have a sudden insight into the patient's problems, without having to analyze things logically.

Through Therapeutic Touch, the practitioner assists the healing process by intentionally directing a life energy that passes through her to the recipient. The practitioner does not use her own energy, but instead acts as a conduit for a universal energy that helps the body to maintain its order. This healing energy is a force that both the practitioner and patient can feel, and that the practitioner directs by following specific steps. These are centering, assessment of the energy flow, balancing the energy, and finally, transferring energy to the person being treated. While the practitioner treats the patient she makes a conscious intent to help.

Centering

To practice Therapeutic Touch effectively, the practitioner must not be distracted by her emotions, or any mental chatter, but should remain focused throughout the entire treatment. This important preparation for Therapeutic Touch is called centering. When the practitioner centers, she withdraws her attention from the external world, and becomes aware of a sense of stillness and peace within. At the same time, she makes an intent to help the recipient.

There is a simple exercise that we teach in our workshops to help participants practice centering.

—Sit quietly in a chair in a comfortable position.
—Close your eyes and become aware of your breathing.
—Focus your attention in the area of your heart.
—Think of something that for you is a symbol of peace—a tree, a mountain, the ocean.
—Think of the peaceful feeling as being inside yourself. Say to yourself, "I am that peace."

Another way to center is to simply become aware of your breathing.

—Inhale and exhale slowly.
—Become aware of the space between breaths.
—Notice the feeling of quiet, almost as if time is suspended.

Dolores Krieger calls this technique "instant centering" because we can use it in any busy situation to immediately quiet ourselves.

Many Therapeutic Touch recipients are sick, and as a result are anxious or in pain. Centering is a tool that allows the Therapeutic Touch practitioner to remain focused on her intent to help the patient, without becoming identified with the recipient's anxiety or emotional turmoil. Because we can easily be affected by another's feelings, the practitioner may experience a patient's fear or pain as a vague anxiety within herself. When the practitioner remains centered, she remains sensitive to her patient's feelings, but is able to keep her own emotions from intruding on the treatment. At the same time, as the practitioner projects peace and quiet to the patient, she keeps from becoming overidentified with the patient's feelings. She is aware of the patient's emotional disturbance, but still remains emotionally and mentally calm. This attitude of the practitioner, which some nurses call "contagious calmness," transfers to the patient, helping him to relax. As we will see in Chapter Five, the ability to relax makes the person being treated more receptive to healing.

The centered practitioner also remains free of anxiety about the results of the treatment. She is able to send healing energy so that the body can use it, but let go of the need for a specific outcome of the treatment. This detachment on the part of a health professional seems unusual, because in most hospitals and clinics, nurses and doctors have specific goals for their patients in mind. These goals relate to their definition of healing, which is usually that of return of function. If a patient has a broken leg, for example, healing of the bone restores the leg's function—the patient will be able to walk again. As we discussed in Chapter Three, although functional return is part of the healing process, there is more. If we consider healing to be an integration of physical, emotional, mental, and creative energies, resulting in the patient's experiencing a sense of wholeness, then healing can take place whether or not there is return of physical function. A cancer patient, for example, may never be cured of cancer, yet can have a satisfying life and make a creative contribution to others. He may also experience a pain-free and peaceful death. These experiences may represent healing for this person, even though the cancer is still present.

When the practitioner has this wider definition of healing, she is able to detach from the outcome of Therapeutic Touch, or any other medical intervention. Although the practitioner has an understandable wish to help the patient improve, her self esteem does not depend on whether or not the patient experiences functional improvement. By attending to the process of the treatment and letting go of the need for a specific outcome, the practitioner remains relaxed and becomes a more effective transmitter of healing energy. The practitioner makes a clear intent to help another, lets go of the need to control the result, and trusts that the patient will use the extra energy to restore order within the body.

Although the practice of Therapeutic Touch requires quieting the emotions and the mind, and setting aside the attachment to outcome, this does not mean that the Therapeutic Touch practitioner must be problem-free. During the treatment, though, she sets aside the usual worries of daily life and is not distracted by her environment. In this frame of mind the practitioner proceeds to the assessment of the patient.

Assessment

In Therapeutic Touch workshops, participants learn to sense the flow of energy within and around the body by using their hands. After the practitioner is quiet, she moves her hands slowly over the surface of the body, about two to three inches above the surface of the skin, while the patient, who is fully dressed, sits comfortably in a chair. The practitioner moves her hands in a downward motion, from head to foot over the patient, first in front and then in back. She is seeking subtle sensations with her hands, to determine where the patient's energy flow changes, where it is blocked, or where the normal smooth rhythm of the energy flow is disrupted.

The Therapeutic Touch practitioner is trained to feel sensations that are not part of our usual daily experience. They are fairly easy to feel, however, and in our one day workshops, which by now have trained thousands of people, there is rarely anyone who is unable to feel this energy flow.

Most people feel healthy energy as a soft warmth under their hands, almost like a light, gentle stream of water. In areas where the flow of energy is blocked, the warmth suddenly feels cooler, and the sense of motion disappears. Over parts of the body where the energy is flowing slowly, the practitioner usually feels a stickiness, or a sense of pressure under her hands. If a patient has an energy deficit—that is, a place where the energy is low—the practitioner often experiences a pulling sensation when she places her hands over the area. She may also have the sense that warmth is being drawn from her hands as she places them over the area low in energy. Energy deficits often, but not always, correspond to an area where the patient has an actual physical problem, such as an infection, wound, or fracture.

The practitioner should assess the patient quickly and

without undue effort. If the assessment takes too long, and if the practitioner thinks or worries too much about what she is doing, the patient often begins to feel a sense of heaviness or pressure, sometimes around the head. Because the energy of the practitioner and the patient is connected, the patient may sense the practitioner's performance anxiety or forced concentration, and feel vaguely uncomfortable.

The assessment is both an external and an internal process. During this phase of treatment, the practitioner works with her hands to pick up cues about the patient's energy, but it is equally important that the internal state of the practitioner be receptive, quiet, and open, so that she receives information with the whole self, not just the hands. In Therapeutic Touch workshops, we suggest that the students record mental impressions about their patients, and then move to the next impression, without making judgments about what they are sensing. With experience, many practitioners become aware intuitively of their patient's physical and emotional problems. Sometimes they will see a mental picture of where the energy flow is blocked, or sense the patients' feelings about their illness. One nurse, who has practiced Therapeutic Touch for several years, describes the internal nature of assessment:

When I first learned to assess a patient, it felt as if my hands went through someone else's energy field, and that I was touching something that had nothing to do with me. At some point, I realized that the assessment had gone from being an over-there process, to an in-here process. Whenever I assessed, although I was using my hands as an outward mode of assessment, at least as much of the information I got came from mental images about the patient's physical condition or emotional state.

Over twenty years of experience with Therapeutic Touch has taught us that the locations of energy imbalances deter-

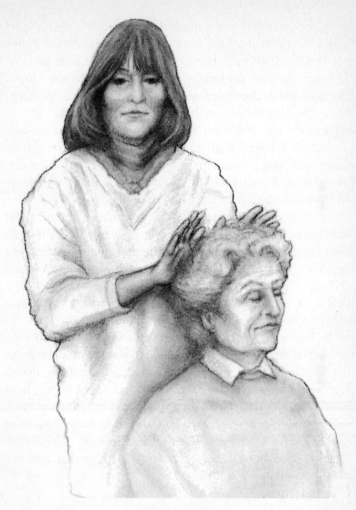

Assessment

mined by assessing the body do not necessarily correlate with the location of the patient's symptoms. Often minor aches and pains in one location are associated with congested or blocked energy in another. In treating patients with headaches, for example, practitioners often find the energy partially blocked around the neck and shoulders. Patients with sore throats often have energy congestion over their throats. However, the extreme fatigue which is part of the sore throat may manifest as decreased energy in the area of the low back. When the practitioner mobilizes the energy in the area of congestion, the symptom in the other location often improves, or disappears altogether. At times, the location of energy imbalance does correlate with the location of a diseased organ. Patients with a stomach ulcer, for example, often have a disruption of the usual rhythm of their energy over the upper abdomen. Patients with infections or fractures will often have a deficit of energy over the area affected. Although there can be correlation between medical diagnosis and energy field imbalances, Therapeutic Touch is a method of describing what is happening with the whole system of the patient. It is not the same as medical diagnosis, which is a highly complex system of classification.

The beginning practitioner will sometimes be able to validate her findings because they will correlate with a symptom or complaint of the person being treated. Or the patient's improvement after the treatment will confirm the energy field assessment. Working with an experienced practitioner for a long period of time is an excellent way of becoming adept at assessing the energy field. The beginner receives valuable instruction, and has the opportunity to compare her findings with someone more skilled.

Balancing the Energy Field

After the practitioner is centered and focused on the treatment, and after she assesses the energy flow, she begins to balance the energy field. This helps the patient's energy to flow freely, and reestablishes its characteristic rhythm.

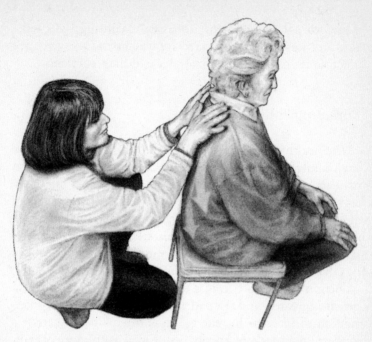

Balancing the Energy Field

While balancing the patient's energy, the practitioner moves the hands downward in long sweeping motions, and at the same time projects a feeling of calm toward the patient. Gentle downward strokes comfort and relax the patient, as long as the practitioner works rhythmically. If she does not, she will disrupt the unique rhythm of the patient's energy flow and as a result he may feel light-headed, anxious, or vaguely uncomfortable.

Balancing the energy field promotes a physiological relaxation response: The patient's breathing slows, and his hands and feet begin to warm, as more blood flows to his extremities. As we will discuss in more detail in Chapter Five, the relaxation response promotes the healing process by stimulating the immune system, which is responsible for the body's main defense against many illnesses. Balancing the energy also prepares the patient to receive healing energy which the practitioner directs in the final phase of the treatment.

Directing Energy

The healthy person continually exchanges energy with the environment, and with others. When we are healthy we experience this exchange as vitality—literally feeling full of energy. During illness our energy becomes depleted, and our ability to take in energy from others and from our surroundings decreases. We experience this relative energy deficit as fatigue, irritability, or pain. In a minor illness like a cold or flu, the energy deficit is small, and sufficient rest and stress reduction will restore it. In a more serious illness, the energy deficit is greater, and the patient often requires outside intervention to increase his energy. In chronic illness, there is a long-standing lack of energy, associated with more chronic obstruction to energy flow. For this reason chronic illness usually requires treatment with Therapeutic Touch, as an adjunct to regular medical care, over a long period of time, while acute problems often respond rapidly.

During a Therapeutic Touch treatment, after the practitioner has assessed the energy imbalances, and reestablished healthy flow, she transmits energy to the patient. This boosts the patient's life energy, and helps him to repattern it in a way that promotes healing. While directing energy to a patient, the practitioner moves her hands over the areas of the body that she has identified to be low in energy. While doing this, she thinks of the healing energy as flowing through her, into the patient. Some practitioners symbolize this energy flow by imagining a waterfall or a white light flowing through them, into the patient. The practitioner should conceptualize the energy as *moving*. Because the patient is a dynamic system of energy flow, when the practitioner imagines the energy as moving into the patient, the treatment is more effective. While the practitioner is directing energy to a specific place in the patient's body, she makes a clear mental picture of the patient as well, and thinks of his body, mind, emotions, and intuition as working together.

Some practitioners, while directing energy, project a specific color to the patient. They think of a stream of colored light entering the patient's body, flooding the system, and exiting through the feet. Clinical experience demonstrates that the most helpful color to project, besides white, is cobalt blue—the purplish blue color seen in stained glass windows. This shade has a sedating effect. It will calm the anxious person and decrease pain. When cobalt blue is used to relieve pain, the practitioner thinks of it as flowing gently through the brain, which contains the centers that perceive pain, and then flooding the part of the body that is the source of the pain.

Although we teach Therapeutic Touch in steps—centering, assessment, balancing the energy, and directing energy—in reality the patient's energy pattern is constantly changing during the treatment. As the practitioner releases congested energy and fills up energy deficits, the energy field becomes smoother and begins to expand. To remain aware of the changes taking place, the practitioner continues to reassess the patient as she transfers energy. As she finishes directing energy, the practitioner balances the energy field once again. She smoothes the energy in a downward motion starting at the head and ending at the feet, while thinking of the patient as healthy and integrated, and of his body as orderly and balanced.

Most Therapeutic Touch treatments last from ten to fifteen minutes. When the treatment is drawing to a close, the practitioner often gets an intuitive or subjective sense that it is time to stop. Once the treatment is completed, the patient

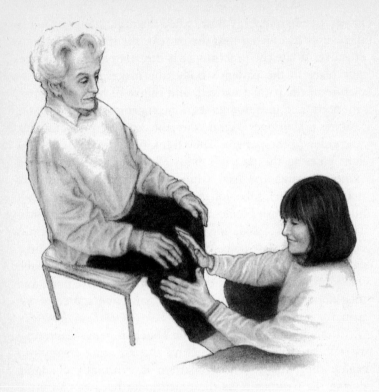

Directing Energy

should sit quietly for at least ten minutes, if possible. Experience demonstrates that there are more long lasting results if the patient's system has time to assimilate the energy before he resumes his usual activity.

The Patient's Experience

During the Therapeutic Touch treatment, the recipient sits quietly in a chair, or lies on his back in bed if he is too sick, or in too much pain, to sit up. As the practitioner balances his energy, the patient relaxes. Sometimes he feels sensations of warmth or cold in the areas where the practitioner is working. Other times, the patient feels very little. The experience of the patient has no effect on the outcome of the treatment. The patient may relax and be fully aware of where the practitioner is working with his hands; yet after the treatment there may be very little change in the original complaint or condition. Or the patient may feel nothing, yet will later find that his original problem has improved markedly.

Many patients find that a Therapeutic Touch treatment increases their vitality and sense of well-being, and sometimes lends insight into difficulties they are facing. Because many physical problems also have an emotional component, some patients find that after treatment, feelings arise that relate to significant life events. Sometimes these feelings are about present situations, but more commonly are associated with the past. These effects seem to be independent of whether or not the treatment relieves the patient's physical problems.

One patient, Robert, asked for Therapeutic Touch to supplement his regular medical therapy for asthma. Five years before he came for treatment he began to experience wheezing and shortness of breath from time to time. His symptoms became more severe and more frequent, and his doctors did not know why. After several Therapeutic Touch treatments, Robert began to grieve the loss of his brother, who had died about two years before his asthma began. As he experienced the extent of his loss, his symptoms began to improve.

Another patient, Alison, requested Therapeutic Touch treatment for low back pain, which had become chronic since the birth of her first child several months before. During her treatment, Alison realized that she felt overwhelmed and sometimes lonely in her role as a new mother. She was able to talk about her feelings with the Therapeutic Touch practitioner, and together they discussed the steps Alison could take to get more support from friends and family.

If the patient experiences emotional distress during the Therapeutic Touch treatment, the practitioner can best help by remaining calm, and projecting a sense of quiet toward the recipient. The practitioner should remain nonjudgmental and supportive and allow the patient to express his feelings. If the patient's emotional problems are complex, or if he is overwhelmed by his feelings, the Therapeutic Touch practitioner should refer him for appropriate professional help.

The Practitioner's Experience

There is a remarkable similarity in the experience of Therapeutic Touch practitioners. In 1990, Dr. Patricia Heidt published the results of a qualitative study that described the experiences of nurses and patients during Therapeutic Touch treatments. Seven nurses participated, each of whom had practiced Therapeutic Touch for at least three years. Each nurse selected a patient willing to be observed during the Therapeutic Touch treatment, and interviewed afterwards. All of the nurses described a similar experience. As they prepared for treatment, the nurses quieted themselves emotionally and mentally and became aware of what they called a universal life energy. They made an intent to open themselves to this life energy and direct it to their patients. One of the nurses in the study said:

> I get a sense of my own wholeness. It's hard to say just what the experience is. It's my connectedness to life, to the source of life. I try to be aware that it is welling up in me and flowing through me. [1]

During the assessment of the patient's energy field, the nurses became attuned to the flow of life energy within their patients. One nurse describes sensing with her patient a "unity and harmony."[2] While balancing the patient's energy, the nurses described the pain or disease of the patient as a "block" in energy flow—a place within the energy field where the energy seemed stuck and was not flowing freely. After they removed these impediments to energy flow, the nurses transferred energy to their patients. They experienced themselves as opening up to a universal energy flow, and directing this toward their patients, at a specific place in the patient's body where it was needed. The nurses sensed their patients "pulling in" the energy.

Dr. Dolores Krieger has also studied extensively the practitioner's experience during Therapeutic Touch. After collecting data for several years, she devised a questionnaire called the "Subjective Experience of Therapeutic Touch Scale" (SETTS). She used it to determine if there were specific experiences that could predict the length of time the practitioner had used Therapeutic Touch. She discovered that most experienced practitioners feel physically relaxed and integrated during Therapeutic Touch treatments, and sometimes experience a heightened awareness of their senses. Experienced practitioners also report increased feelings of calm, and a greater sensitivity to the problems of the patient. They usually feel somewhat detached from their own feelings during the Therapeutic Touch treatment, and more aware of the feelings of their patients. Practitioners feel empathy for their patients, whether or not they like them as individuals.

As practitioners become more adept, there are two significant experiences that they have more frequently. They experience a sense of the unity underlying the seeming diversity of life, and their intuitive abilities expand. During Therapeutic Touch treatments, they become more aware of the connection between themselves and their patients. They are less conscious of their separateness, although they still maintain their own focus of awareness. With time, this sense of unity becomes stronger, affecting the practitioners' other life experiences as well. They become more aware of the interconnectedness of all forms of life, and the commonality of the human experience. Most practitioners of Therapeutic Touch feel a responsibility not simply to oneself and family, but a larger imperative to contribute to the whole. Dolores Krieger believes that eventually the practitioner begins to experience herself and others as "human energy fields that flow through life together." The space between people becomes an extension of those fields and is experienced not "as a place of separation but . . . as an avenue connecting people."[3]

During a Therapeutic Touch treatment the practitioner sometimes becomes aware of the patient's problems in an intuitive way. Although she does not abandon her ability to think logically, her intuition is enhanced. If we remember that during the treatment the practitioner and patient for the moment are energetically linked, it is not surprising that the practitioner may become aware of information about the patient's problem without the need for conversation. This knowing through the intuition is separate but complementary to our usual symbolic or logical way of knowing. Intuitive knowledge is direct and immediate and results from the knower's unity with what is known. Our logical way of looking at the world, on the other hand, requires that the knower separate himself from whatever he is analyzing, and then be able to represent it in abstract symbols, such as language or mathematical concepts. The Therapeutic Touch practitioner uses both logic and intuition in working with her patients. Although intuition may make her aware of things that she would not ordinarily know, it is not a substitute for discrimination. The practitioner's critical judgment is a partner to her intuition.

As the practitioner's intuition becomes more developed, she becomes more self-aware. She identifies less with her transient feelings and thoughts and more with a sense of inner peace that is the foundation of her identity. The development of intuition also makes the practitioner mindful of the wholeness that underlies a diverse and seemingly disordered world. Not only is the practitioner more aware of her own integration, but she perceives the underlying wholeness in her patient, despite the presence of disease or disability.

Eventually, the practitioner's development of intuition begins to affect not only her Therapeutic Touch treatments, but her daily life as well. She becomes more creative, and more self-directed. Janet Macrae describes this in her book, *Therapeutic Touch, A Practical Guide*:

> . . . this intuitiveness will not be limited to your Therapeutic Touch treatments, but will begin to permeate all your actions . . . you will probably become more certain about the direction and meaning of your life as a whole. For it is this intuitive inner directedness that gives us our sense of intrinsic identity or completeness as individuals: the sense that we are not living superficially, responding to external pressures alone, but are also in touch with the creative insight of our own inner nature.[4]

It is not only the patient, then, who benefits from Therapeutic Touch, but the practitioner, too, reaching out with intent to help, transforms herself as well.

5

The Effects of
Therapeutic Touch

IN HER TWENTY years of experience with Therapeutic Touch, Dolores Krieger has traveled and taught extensively throughout the country. She has had the opportunity to treat and observe thousands of patients. In her most recent book, *Accepting Your Power to Heal*, she describes three effects of Therapeutic Touch that she considers to be the most reliable. From her perspective, which many other practitioners share, the most common effect of Therapeutic Touch is rapid relaxation, which is accompanied by the patient's experiencing a feeling of well-being. The next most reliable results are the relief of pain and an acceleration of the body's natural healing process.[1]

Therapeutic Touch and Relaxation

Frequently, anxiety is a companion of illness. Except in circumstances where illness is mild, most of us feel anxiety about its outcome. If we are not able to perform our usual activities, we often become worried about our responsibilities at work or at home. If we need to make minor adjustments in our lives, we often experience some stress related to change alone. In cases of serious illness, such as cancer or HIV related disease, we may have more profound anxiety about our ability to be self-sufficient. Fear of disability or death may compound physical suffering, and add enormously to the burden of illness. The anxiety that accompanies physical disease often becomes a source of constant stress. It can interfere with the body's healing process, because it deprives us of rest. During sleep, the body's repair processes are stimulated, and physical regeneration occurs.

Nurses who practice Therapeutic Touch use it widely for the relief of anxiety, often in the hospital setting where patients are seriously ill. In addition, psychotherapists sometimes use it as an adjunct to their counseling practices. In both situations it has been effective in calming and relaxing the recipient. Most practitioners find that their patients relax visibly a few minutes after the Therapeutic Touch treatment begins. As the treatment progresses they exhibit even deeper relaxation, and actual physical changes occur. The skin becomes warmer and slightly flushed, the temperature of the hands and feet increases, breathing rate slows, and the pitch of the voice lowers.

These physical changes are similar to those listed by Herbert Benson, a Harvard physician and researcher, who, in 1974, first described what he called the "relaxation response." Benson pointed out that the relaxation response consists of specific physical changes that are the opposite of those that comprise the body's response to stress.[2] During deep relaxation, the heart rate decreases and breathing rate slows. The pupils constrict and the skeletal muscles relax. If researchers test a deeply relaxed individual in a laboratory, they find that his oxygen consumption is reduced, and the amount of lactate in his blood is decreased. These results show that during relaxation the body's metabolism slows down.

The relaxation response is important for health because it serves as an antidote to the fight-or-flight response that occurs when we are under stress. The fight-or-flight response is largely controlled by the sympathetic nervous system, and describes a series of physical changes that prepare the body to handle threats to survival. If we experience an immediate threat, our pupils dilate, and our blood flows primarily to the head and trunk of the body, away from the hands and feet. Our breathing becomes more rapid and shallow, and our heart rate speeds up. The large muscles of our body contract. These physiological changes prepare the threatened individual to fight and survive bodily injury which results, or to flee the situation.

The fight-or-flight response is an important adaptation that ensures survival. In and of itself it is beneficial, if the stress that elicits it is short-lived. In fact, some recent studies show that short-term psychological stress causes a temporary increase in the numbers of natural killer cells present in the blood.[3] These cells are part of the body's immune defense. They destroy foreign invaders and cancer cells. Researchers at the University of California at Los Angeles found that survivors of the 1987 Los Angeles earthquake had an increase in natural killer cells measured in their blood when technicians drew it two to four hours after the disaster.[4] Scientists are not yet sure how these changes measured in blood tests actually affect our day-to-day health. One implication, though, is that short-term stress transiently improves the body's ability to defend itself against disease.

Unremitting stress, however, sets the stage for the occurrence of a variety of health problems. In our fast-paced world, most of us experience stress daily. Unfortunately, the difficulties related to our jobs or family life are not necessarily subject to easy resolution. Fight-or-flight responses may not be appropriate, and unless we know how to manage our stress, it becomes chronic.

During stress, the cortex of the adrenal gland secretes cortisol. This hormone, in the short term, prepares the body to cope with emergency situations. Cortisol causes retention of salt and water by the body, which raises the blood pressure. It also stimulates the liver to make glucose, so that ready fuel is available if an individual needs to act rapidly. These are both useful adaptations for someone who is threatened with physical injury, such as a soldier going into combat. For someone who is under long-term psychological stress, however, high levels of blood cortisol may contribute to many of the illnesses that we consider "psychosomatic." For example, increased cortisol production has been implicated as one factor in the development of stress ulcers, and plays some role in the development of certain forms of high blood pressure.[5] One study, done by Mustafa al'Absi at the University of Oklahoma Health Sciences Center, demonstrated that individuals with borderline high blood pressure produce more cortisol in response to doing a mentally stressful task than do individuals with normal blood pressure.[6]

There is also evidence that suggests that chronic stress depresses the functioning of the immune system. Researchers studied sixty-four dental students under academic stress, and found that an immunoglobulin in their saliva, Ig-A, was significantly lower in periods of stress.[7] Immunoglobulins are antibodies that recognize and destroy specific bacteria or viruses. They are made by B cells, a specific cell of the immune system. Ig-A is present in body fluids and is the first line of defense against foreign invaders.

Janice Kiecolt-Glaser, a psychologist at Ohio State University College of Medicine, has studied the effects of chronic stress on family members who were caregivers of patients with Alzheimer's disease.[8] She found the caregivers to be more mentally depressed than the noncaregivers with whom she compared them. In laboratory tests, they had fewer total T cells and helper T cells. T cells are lymphocytes that are particularly critical in the body's defense against viruses, fungal infection, and cancer. Helper T cells turn on the immune response. Suppressor T cells turn it off when it is no longer needed.

Because the effects of chronic stress may be detrimental to our health, researchers have been interested in exploring whether or not the relaxation response can ward off its effects. Some of their results demonstrate that because the relaxation response is physiologically opposite from the changes induced by chronic stress, it can be helpful in promoting health.

There are many ways of inducing a relaxation response. Herbert Benson, in his original paper, describes four conditions that are usually necessary in order for an individual to experience a relaxation response.[9] The person should be in a quiet environment, without distraction. He should be in a physically comfortable position. He need not make an effort to relax, but should have a passive attitude. He also needs to shift from what Benson calls "logical, externally-oriented thought." One tool that aids this shift is for the person to narrow his awareness of the environment by focusing attention on a specific object in his surroundings, or repeating silently a sound or phrase.

There are several different techniques that combine these basic features, and result in a physiological relaxation response. Some of these are meditation, autogenic training, yoga, and progressive relaxation. Of these, both autogenic training and progressive relaxation are more commonly used in the Western system of health care. Autogenic training developed from the practice of hypnosis for relaxation. In its most commonly used form, patients use self-suggestion to achieve physiological relaxation. Through autogenic training, a person learns to induce relaxation through a series of exercises that he practices daily. By passive concentration, instead of active trying, he practices feeling his arms and legs as heavy and warm. He also concentrates on his heartbeat being calm and regular, and his breathing slow and relaxed.[10]

The technique of progressive relaxation is a method for relaxing skeletal muscles deeply. This is one of the most common methods used in the United States, and was developed by Edmund Jacobson. It is based on his theory that mental anxiety and muscular relaxation cannot coexist. Jacobson believed that muscles are set into patterns of tension when we mentally anticipate or rehearse anxiety-producing events. Through simple exercises, subjects practice both contracting and relaxing their muscles in order to develop an awareness of the sensation of relaxation. By being able to control the contraction of muscles, the individual practicing progressive relaxation can decrease his anxiety as well.

There have been several studies that have examined the effect of the relaxation response on the immune system. In these studies, the subjects used a variety of relaxation techniques, including progressive relaxation, hypnosis, and biofeedback assisted relaxation. In ten studies, done between 1985 and 1990, the most significant finding has been that relaxation techniques increase Ig-A antibody in saliva, and increase the activity of natural killer cells.[11] These results suggest that the relaxation response may enhance our ability to fight disease. However, there still remain many unanswered questions about the relationship between physiological relaxation and health. Although laboratory tests may show that relaxation enhances the immune system, scientists have not clearly established whether an increase in immune cells in the patient's blood also translates to preventing illness in an individual.

As mentioned earlier, Therapeutic Touch practitioners notice that patients feel very relaxed during treatment. Most patients say, "This is so relaxing," or "I feel so peaceful." At the same time, patients exhibit some of the signs of physiological relaxation—warmth and flushing of the skin, and warming of the extremities. This observation led to some attempts to establish whether or not Therapeutic Touch could induce physiological changes that researchers could measure in a laboratory.

In 1979 Dolores Krieger, Erik Peper, and Sonia Ancoli studied Dolores Krieger, acting as Therapeutic Touch practitioner, in a laboratory at the Langley Porter Neuropsychiatric Institute at UCLA.[12] The purpose of the study was to gain information about the physiological state of the practitioner during Therapeutic Touch. At the same time, the researchers measured the physiological response of three patients during their Therapeutic Touch treatments. The researchers recorded the patients' brain waves (EEG), muscle tension (EMG), and the ability of their skin to conduct electrical current (GSR). They also monitored their heart rates and temperatures. There was no significant change for the patients' electromyographic tracings, their galvanic skin response, heart rates, or temperatures. This differs from the results of most other techniques that elicit deep relaxation, which cause an increase in galvanic skin response, and a decrease in heart rate. However, the patients studied by Krieger, Peper, and Ancoli did have electroencephalographic tracings that demonstrated high amplitude alpha waves in abundance—a sign of being in a relaxed state.

Because the sample of patients studied was small, the researchers drew no firm conclusions. However, because of the patients' brain wave changes, the study did suggest that Therapeutic Touch could produce a relaxation response. This led to further research. In 1981, psychotherapist Dr. Patricia Heidt published the results of a study that examined the effects of Therapeutic Touch on the anxiety level of patients hospitalized for cardiovascular disease.[13] Dr. Heidt studied ninety patients. Thirty received Therapeutic Touch and thirty received casual touch, which consisted of a nurse taking pulses on the hands and feet. Thirty other patients received no touch. Instead, they had a nurse sit and talk with them for five minutes.

Dr. Heidt measured the anxiety level of the patients with a standardized measure of anxiety called the A-State Self-Evaluation Questionnaire, developed by Speilberger, Gorusch, and Lushene in 1970 as a tool for measuring a person's anxiety at a specific time. Each patient filled out this form both before and after treatment. Dr. Heidt discovered that the patients receiving Therapeutic Touch reported a significant decrease in subjective anxiety after their treatments.

In l982, Dr. Janet Quinn followed this study with another. Dr. Quinn studied sixty patients on the cardiovascular unit of a large hospital.[14] She divided them into two groups. One group received Therapeutic Touch, without any physical contact made by the practitioner. A second group received a mimic Therapeutic Touch treatment, which untrained observers could not differentiate from the real treatment. The patients reported their anxiety level before and after treatment. They used the same self-evaluation questionnaire as did the subjects in Dr. Heidt's study.

The group receiving Therapeutic Touch and the group receiving the mimic treatment both had decreases in their anxiety levels after treatment. However, the patients in the group receiving Therapeutic Touch had a more dramatic and significant decrease in their anxiety level after treatment.

In neither Dr. Heidt's study nor Dr. Quinn's did the researchers use electronic monitoring to determine if Therapeutic Touch treatments caused physiological relaxation. In both of these studies the researchers believed that the monitoring itself could be upsetting to hospitalized cardiac patients, and could affect the outcome of the experiment. What the studies do demonstrate is that Therapeutic Touch is effective in inducing *psychologic* relaxation—a lessening of feelings of anxiety in the patients who received Therapeutic Touch.

In an attempt to find out if Therapeutic Touch could elicit physiological relaxation, Gretchen Randolph, in 1979, studied its effects on sixty healthy female college students.[15] Dr. Randolph designed the study to determine if Therapeutic Touch affected the anxiety level of the students, when they were treated during a stressful situation. Researchers divided the students into two groups. Thirty students received Therapeutic Touch while watching a disturbing movie. The other thirty received a mimic Therapeutic Touch treatment, performed by a nurse who did not know the technique. Researchers electronically monitored both groups to determine if they had any changes in muscle tension, skin temperature, and the ability of the skin to conduct current.

To determine whether Therapeutic Touch reduced anxiety, this study relied only on objective findings, not on whether or not the subject felt relaxed. Dr. Randolph did not detect any significant difference in response between the two groups. There are two factors that may have played a role in her lack of results. The practitioners administered brief Therapeutic Touch treatments, lasting only five minutes. This is an unusually short time in which to be able to expect any effects. In addition, Dr. Randolph's subjects were healthy people. Some earlier studies on healing, done by Dr. Grad, suggest that researchers see more pronounced effects of treatment in subjects who are sick. When they study healthy people, the results are not as dramatic.

Therapeutic Touch clearly is able to produce subjective relaxation. It also produces clinically observable signs of physiological relaxation—warming and flushing of skin, slowing of breathing rate. As yet, though, there is no reliable and reproducible evidence that it provides the same electronically monitored physiological changes that scientists see in some other methods that produce a relaxation response. Despite this, some recent studies do suggest that, like other relaxation techniques, Therapeutic Touch may improve the functioning of the immune system. Janet Quinn, now a professor of Nursing at the University of Colorado Health Sciences Center in Denver, examined the effects of Therapeutic Touch on the immune systems of grieving patients.[16]

Dr. Quinn studied four patients who were deeply grieving after the death of a relative. A Therapeutic Touch practitioner treated each patient once a day for seven days. Technicians drew blood from the patients before the treatment, to establish a baseline. They then drew blood after the treatment. For all four patients, there was a drop of 18% in their suppressor T cell count. As mentioned earlier, suppressor T cells are responsible for regulating the immune response. Their job is to turn off antibody production. A drop in suppressor T cells suggests an enhancement of immunity.

Although this study is promising, because its sample size is small we need to use caution in interpreting its results. Another recent study, however, funded by the National Institutes of Health, also suggests that Therapeutic Touch may enhance immunity. Dr. Melodie Olson, at the Medical University of South Carolina, studied the effects of Therapeutic Touch on twenty highly stressed nursing and medical students. Dr. Olson and other researchers treated ten students with Therapeutic Touch for three days before they took professional board exams. Another ten students received no treatment. When the students' blood was drawn, those who had received Therapeutic Touch for three days had significantly increased the levels of immunoglobulins in their blood, compared with a baseline value drawn before the study began. These immunoglobulins—Ig-A, Ig-G and Ig-M—play specific roles in fighting infection. The group that received no Therapeutic Touch had no change in their immunoglobulin levels.

Dr. Olson's study shows that, by increasing the numbers of circulating antibodies in the patient's blood, Therapeutic Touch affects the body in ways that we can measure scientifically. Scientists have yet to determine whether increased antibody levels also translate to improved health for patients. Nevertheless, this study points the way for further research to establish the role of Therapeutic Touch in enhancing immunity.

Therapeutic Touch may also affect the immune system by helping the recipient to experience and understand his emotions. The relaxation associated with Therapeutic Touch promotes emotional release. When the patient is quiet and calm, feelings sometimes arise that may relate to events in his present or past. Sometimes this occurs during treatment or sometimes within a few days after treatment. Scientists are beginning to understand that emotional expression affects the functioning of the immune system. Psychologists Ann Futterman, Margaret Kemeny, and their colleagues evaluated the effect of emotional expression on the cells of the immune system.[17] The researchers studied sixteen actors who were instructed to experience specific emotional states. The psychologists asked them to improvise emotions of relaxed happiness, euphoria, depression, and agitation, by recalling and acting out events related to their experience. For example, the researchers asked them to remember and improvise a success after a major performance. Technicians drew blood from the actors before they began, in order to determine a baseline value for their immune cells. They drew blood again twenty minutes after the start of the improvisation, and then again after a twenty-minute recovery time, to see if there were changes in the numbers of immune cells and their ability to function. Researchers compared the results from the actors with those of a control group, who read out loud from magazines. Their reading material was emotionally neutral.

The actors expressing emotion, whether positive or negative, had a higher percentage of natural killer cells in their blood, and the cells were more active. After twenty minutes, the cells returned to their baseline level. The study suggests that emotional expression, regardless of whether the person is happy or sad, stimulates the immune system temporarily.

In another study, researchers asked fifty healthy students to write about personal traumatic events for twenty minutes each day, for four days.[18] This activity enhanced the students' immune response. Not only did some of their immune cells function more effectively when tested in the laboratory, but the students also had fewer visits to their health service. The researchers conducting the study believe that confronting the emotions associated with the traumatic events may lead to better health.

Since the research described above demonstrates that emotional release has some effect on immune functioning, we can hypothesize that this would be true for patients receiving Therapeutic Touch, as well. However, practitioners have yet to study the effects of Therapeutic Touch–induced emotional expression on the immune system. We need further study to understand how emotional expression affects our immunity.

Therapeutic Touch and Pain Relief

Pain is a universal human experience, and a signal to the body that its integrity is somehow threatened and corrective measures need to be taken. Placing a hand on a hot stove hurts, and this signals us that thermal injury to the skin is beginning. Pain sends the message to remove our hand to protect it from burning. In the same way, serious chest or abdominal pain warns us of a medical problem needing attention. Although pain causes suffering, it is a valuable mechanism that gives us information about the functioning of our bodies.

Physicians divide pain into two categories—acute and chronic. Acute pain has a clear, identifiable cause. It is usually present for a short time (hours, instead of days) and when the patient takes medication, it usually relieves the pain. Relaxation techniques, such as hypnosis, biofeedback, and Therapeutic Touch all relieve acute pain, at least partially. These techniques help to relieve the anxiety that accompanies pain. Since anxiety plays a role in how the patient perceives pain, relieving anxiety will also diminish the sensation of pain.

Therapeutic Touch practitioners have successfully treated patients with acute pain from a variety of causes. During the treatment, the practitioner thinks of sending energy into the area that is painful, in order to break up the congested energy that sometimes accompanies pain. Many practitioners imagine a cobalt blue light flowing through the patient, flooding the brain, which registers pain sensation, and continuing throughout the body to bathe the area that causes pain. This practice relaxes the patient and usually reduces the pain in the affected area. The pain may be relieved during the treatment, and relief can last for up to several hours.

In 1986, Elizabeth Keller, a nurse practitioner in Texas, and Virginia Bzdek, a professor of Nursing at the University of Missouri, studied sixty patients with headache.[19] The researchers wanted to see if Therapeutic Touch would be effective in relieving their pain. They divided the patients into two groups. One group received Therapeutic Touch and the other received a mimic Therapeutic Touch treatment. Keller and Bdzek used a form, called the McGill Melzack Pain Questionnaire, to evaluate whether the patients responded to treatment. This questionnaire has been widely used to assess pain relief in many kinds of clinical studies. The patients in this study filled it out both before and after treatment.

Therapeutic Touch reduced headache in 90% of the patients. The average pain reduction for these patients was 70%. The mimic treatment reduced pain in 80%, but the average pain reduction for these patients was only 37%. During the four hours after treatment, only five patients treated with Therapeutic Touch needed medication to relieve their headaches. In the other group, fifteen patients used other treatments to relieve their headaches.

Nurses, massage therapists, physical therapists, and some physicians have used Therapeutic Touch successfully in the treatment of chronic pain, but its use for this problem has not been studied scientifically. Chronic pain is much more complex than acute pain, because it can be harder for physicians to determine its causes, and more challenging to treat. Since there are often many factors contributing to chronic pain, it is more difficult for researchers to study.

Chronic pain falls into two categories. Chronic malignant pain is usually the result of progressive, identifiable disease, such as cancer or serious arthritis. Physicians can usually pinpoint the cause of this kind of pain. Medication often takes it away, but some patients may require larger and larger doses for relief.

A second type of chronic pain is chronic nonmalignant pain, which is often the most difficult for patients to tolerate and for doctors to treat. By definition, to be considered chronic, it must exist for greater than three months. Usually no clear cause for the pain is apparent. Patients suffering from chronic nonmalignant pain often become depressed and despondent because of a lack of diagnosis, and the unremitting nature of their discomfort.

Although doctors and nurses approach pain scientifically, for the patient, it is a highly personal experience. Although we perceive pain physically, it is also an emotional and mental experience. Pain affects our thoughts and feelings, which in turn have an impact on how we interpret it.

The most common emotion associated with pain, whether acute or chronic, is anxiety. The person with pain often fears it will become more severe. If he is temporarily pain-free, he worries about its return. A patient with serious illness feels apprehensive about bodily deterioration that the pain represents. A patient who has chronic pain often experiences an erosion of his self-confidence. He feels limited in what he can do, for fear of increasing the pain. He may doubt that the pain will ever go away, and eventually, if it persists long enough, he becomes helpless and hopeless, not only about the pain, but about other aspects of his life as well. He may become chronically frustrated, because the limitations caused by the pain fall short of his ideal for himself.

Eventually chronic pain may become part of a person's self-image, and this leads to identification with pain. Since the patient has difficulty remembering a time without pain, he also finds it impossible to imagine a future without it. A person with chronic pain may become more and more turned inward and focused on his distress. He may feel overwhelmed by his pain, and find it difficult to relate to friends and family. Social relationships and work suffer as a result.

Therapeutic Touch is useful in helping people with chronic pain, but needs to be used as a tool to help mobilize the self-healing capacities of the pain sufferer. Jane Williams is a physiotherapist in Vancouver, B.C. In her work with chronic pain patients, she integrates Therapeutic Touch with both physical therapy and massage therapy. She describes her approach to patients with this problem:

Many patients come to me who have been living busy lives, in which they are overinvolved and overextended. Suddenly they are injured in an auto accident, for example, and find that they are not the same person as before. Their lives have become more shut off because of pain. They tend to close in and focus on the pain. Their social lives and work lives may come to a halt. Although friends and family are often initially supportive, they tend to fall away, as pain becomes chronic and the patient doesn't get better.

I help the patient see that the pain is not necessarily

bad, and that it can provide an opportunity to make some changes. It is important to mobilize the patient's sense of wellness, and to help him set small achievable goals for himself. I try to help the patient find a sense of peace and a connection with his inner self. To assist this I give suggestions for homework. This can be as simple as taking a walk in nature, or spending a few minutes every day thinking of an image that represents peace.

When I treat a chronic pain patient with Therapeutic Touch, he sometimes has temporary pain relief. This experience wakes up a memory of what it is like to be without pain. It helps the patient to see that he is more than the pain, that there is a part of him that can transcend the pain. But, using Therapeutic Touch alone, without helping the patient to mobilize his own resources, can sometimes encourage dependence on the treatment itself. If the patient sees relief solely as coming from outside himself, it can further undermine his self-confidence.

Dora Kunz and Erik Peper, in a paper called "The Pain Process and Strategies for Pain Reduction,"[20] underscore the importance of caretakers helping the patient to mobilize his inner resources. This attitude is based on the belief that within the sick person is a self-healing potential, and that it is possible for the caretaker to reach outward and nurture this potential. Kunz and Peper also offer several suggestions for the patient with chronic pain, who can use them to enhance his ability to help himself. The patient can:

—Learn to direct the focus of his thoughts away from the pain. Attending to the pain often intensifies the perception of pain; focusing on some other activity helps to reduce it.

—Do something, however small, for someone else. This focuses attention away from the pain and energizes the patient.

—Accept the pain, without judging or asking "Why me?" Instead seek solutions that will help solve the problem. Realize that the pain is present *at this moment*, but need not be a part of the future.

A patient suffering chronic pain may find that it affects his relationships with family and friends. He often becomes lost in his sensation of pain, and if his pain persists for any length of time, he can become isolated from family members. If he is angry and frustrated, he further alienates his family. Family members sometimes become frustrated themselves, because they would like to help but don't know how.

Pain sufferers often feel both physically and emotionally drained. Because the pain fatigues the patient, and makes him extremely sensitive, family members can best help by adopting an attitude of quiet caring. If they can remain calm within and help the patient see that their affection continues, the patient will usually feel less isolated. It is best for the family to avoid repetitively asking, "How are you?" Although this is an innocent and often automatic question, it often makes the patient feel like a failure for not having improved. It is more helpful for the family to let the patient know that they enjoy his company, despite his disability.

Some Therapeutic Touch practitioners have trained friends and family members of patients to do Therapeutic Touch. Family members find that this is something they can do to be of help, and as a result feel less frustrated. As they practice Therapeutic Touch, they learn to be quiet and centered within. Family members communicate this sense of inner peace to the sick person, and it helps to relieve his anxiety.

Therapeutic Touch and the Acceleration of Healing

The clinical experience with Therapeutic Touch over the past twenty years teaches us that Therapeutic Touch speeds up the usual process of healing. This does not occur by any magic formula, but is simply the acceleration of the usual process of repair and regeneration that is part of the body's natural healing ability. The effect is most apparent for illnesses that involve wound repair, bone repair, and the body's ability to fight infection.

A remarkable example of wound repair is the case of a woman in her sixties who attended a Therapeutic Touch training session for health professionals on Orcas Island a few years ago. Yvonne attended the workshop as a patient, hoping that Therapeutic Touch could help her. She was a diabetic who also had mild heart disease. Her most serious problem at the time was a skin ulcer on her leg. This is a common complication of serious diabetes and is often difficult to treat. During her weeklong stay on Orcas, practitioners treated her daily with Therapeutic Touch. She also continued her usual medical treatment. After seven days, her skin ulcer was about 60% healed. This is a very rapid rate of improvement for a diabetic skin ulcer, which often takes weeks to months to resolve, even with the best of medical care.

Many nurses who practice Therapeutic Touch on orthopedic units of hospitals report similar experiences in the acceleration of healing of fractures. Patients who are treated with Therapeutic Touch, in addition to their usual orthopedic treatment for fractures, usually show improvement of the X rays sooner than is typical for most patients. Significant improvement after three weeks is the norm. This contrasts with

the usual six weeks that it takes to see adequate bone healing.[21]

In an attempt to scientifically demonstrate whether or not
Therapeutic Touch could accelerate healing, researcher Daniel Wirth evaluated its effect on the rate of wound healing.[22]
He studied forty-four volunteers, each of whom agreed to
have a small uniform surgical wound placed on his arm. Each
day after wounding, each subject would stick his arm
through a circular hole in a wall. The researchers told each
volunteer that they wanted to measure "biopotentials" from
the wound. The patients were unable to see what was happening on the other side of the wall, and at no time did they
have physical contact with anyone. Half of the patients received daily Therapeutic Touch, and half of the patients received no treatment. In fact, there was no one present in the
room where the control patients had placed their arms. At
several stages, a physician, who knew nothing about the experiment, evaluated the wound. He traced the wound size
onto transparent acetate sheets, which researchers then gave
to a technician, who further evaluated wound size.

The results of the study demonstrated that patients receiving Therapeutic Touch healed more quickly than patients receiving no treatment. By the eighth day of the study, the
patients who were treated showed more improvement than
the patients who were not. By day sixteen, the wounds of
thirteen of the twenty-two patients who received Therapeutic
Touch were completely healed. None of the untreated group
were better.

Besides demonstrating that Therapeutic Touch accelerates
wound healing, this study is significant because of its control
for the placebo effect. This effect is a factor in the delivery
of all medical care, including Therapeutic Touch. The act of
treatment itself, regardless of what it is, is partially responsible for the benefits of any treatment. There are many factors
that play a role in the placebo effect. The patient's belief in

the treatment can affect its outcome. The beliefs and attitude of the person delivering the treatment can also make a difference in whether or not the patient responds. In studies on Therapeutic Touch, it is very difficult to eliminate the placebo effect completely, because even if the patient is unaware of whether or not they are receiving Therapeutic Touch, the practitioner always knows. In Daniel Wirth's study, the patients were completely unaware that practitioners were treating them. Because they believed that the researachers were measuring "biopotentials" from the wound, they did not even know the researchers were conducting a study on the rate of healing. The expectations of the patients, then, did not play a role in how fast their wounds healed. And, because they had no known contact with the practitioner, her beliefs and expectation could have little or no effect on them.

Other Effects of Therapeutic Touch

Therapeutic Touch affects the functioning of the body's autonomic nervous system. The autonomic nervous system is divided into sympathetic and parasympathetic branches. Working together, they control many physical processes, including blood pressure, heart rate, sweating, body temperature, bowel function, urinary output, and muscle strength. The autonomic nervous system operates by means of visceral reflexes. Sensory signals, coming from parts of the body, go through the spinal cord and into the brain stem and hypothalamus. In turn, the brain transmits impulses back to the body to regulate its functioning. The autonomic nervous system adjusts on a moment to moment basis, always processing new information, and making changes to maintain health.

Imbalance between sympathetic and parasympathetic function causes a variety of ailments. These include cardiac arrythmias, asthma, and some forms of high blood pressure.

Certain gastrointestinal disorders, for example irritable bowel syndrome (a disorder of bowel motility) and some kinds of diarrhea, are also caused by autonomic nervous system imbalance. In general, physicians consider these problems to be stress related disorders.

Therapeutic Touch has been effective in relieving symptoms associated with these stress related disorders. For example, nurses in emergency rooms use Therapeutic Touch to slow the heart rate and relieve chest pains. They also treat asthmatics, who usually experience improvement in their breathing. We do not completely understand why Therapeutic Touch so reliably affects the autonomic nervous system. It is possible that because the system is rapidly changing and always adjusting to new sensory information that it is more responsive to therapeutic techniques. The autonomic nervous system is also very responsive to medical intervention, for example. The administration of appropriate medication has rapid effect on functions that the autonomic nervous system controls.

In contrast to its effects on the autonomic nervous system, Therapeutic Touch has very little effect on some other kinds of problems. Patients with genetic diseases or congenital disorders may experience some symptom improvement when practitioners treat them with Therapeutic Touch, but their underlying disease is unaffected. In the same way, patients with serious illness such as cancer and HIV often experience relief of pain and other symptoms of their illness, but not necessarily a reversal of their disease.

There are a wide range of other disorders in which Therapeutic Touch has been moderately effective in accelerating healing. These include problems related to the circulation, such as edema, and the musculoskeletal system, such as arthritis. Some thyroid diseases also respond well to Therapeutic Touch. In addition, Therapeutic Touch has been used to relieve pain during labor and delivery. We will discuss in more detail some of the uses of Therapeutic Touch in the second part of this book. Another good source for more complete information on the specific uses of Therapeutic Touch is Dolores Krieger's *Accepting Your Power to Heal: The Personal Practice of Therapeutic Touch*.

As we have noted, relief of pain and anxiety and acceleration of healing provided by Therapeutic Touch make it helpful for people with a wide variety of illnesses. Although research in Therapeutic Touch is at its early stages, results so far suggest that there are specific physical benefits resulting from its use. Just as important, Therapeutic Touch has no harmful side effects. Because recipients feel better with no risk of harm, this treatment can be made available, as we continue to gather information to better understand the contribution Therapeutic Touch makes to healing.

SPECIAL

APPLICATIONS

of

THERAPEUTIC

TOUCH

6

❧❧

Therapeutic Touch with Children

ONE OF THE MOST interesting and effective uses of Therapeutic Touch is with babies and children. Practitioners have successfully used Therapeutic Touch at all stages of early life—during pregnancy, labor, and delivery, and in the care of premature infants. They have also treated older children who are sick, both in and out of the hospital.

Some research shows that Therapeutic Touch calms stressful premature babies, and helps hospitalized older children to relax after anxiety-provoking medical tests or examinations. Other research suggests that Therapeutic Touch improves the parents' relationship at the time of childbirth.

Children usually respond more rapidly to Therapeutic Touch than do adults, and they are often more receptive to treatment. Most children relax after only a few minutes of treatment, and sometimes fall asleep afterwards. For these reasons, there are special considerations in using Therapeutic Touch with children, which are described at the chapter's end.

Therapeutic Touch During Pregnancy, Labor, and Delivery

In 1984, Dolores Krieger published the results of a study that examined the effects of Therapeutic Touch when used in conjunction with Lamaze training for childbirth preparation.[1] Dr. Krieger randomly selected sixty couples, all of whom were expecting their first child. Thirty couples prepared for childbirth with Lamaze training only, and served as the control group for the study. The other thirty couples comprised the experimental group. Experienced practitioners trained the husbands in this group to practice Therapeutic Touch on their wives two to three times a week during the last twelve weeks of pregnancy.

The researchers postulated that the use of Therapeutic Touch in childbirth preparation would enhance marital satisfaction and decrease anxiety at the time of labor and delivery. To measure marital satisfaction, they used the Interpersonal Conflict Scale, a questionnaire that the couples completed both before and after delivery. To measure anxiety, the researchers asked the couples to fill out the State-Trait Anxiety Inventory, which measures underlying anxiety, as well as anxiety at any given moment.

When Dr. Krieger compared the anxiety levels of both groups at the end of the study, there was no difference. Both the group who used Therapeutic Touch and the group who used Lamaze alone reported low anxiety both before the study began and after delivery. Dr. Krieger concluded that for the couples in the study the birth of their first child was an event they anticipated happily and was not anxiety-producing. The study did demonstrate, however, that couples who used Therapeutic Touch experienced enhanced marital satisfaction after delivery, compared with the couples using

Lamaze alone. When researchers analyzed the data, they found that the ability to perceive a partner's feelings and the ability to communicate were the best predictors of the couples' marital satisfaction.

While for most families the birth of the first child is a joyous event, it requires that both parents learn new roles and adjust to the presence of a demanding newcomer. These changes take place when lack of rest and irregular sleep leave parents chronically fatigued. Therapeutic Touch, because it enhanced the couples' sensitivity and improved their communication, played a role in easing their adjustment to parenthood. In addition, many men who treated their wives in the study reported that after practicing Therapeutic Touch, they felt a more personal connection to their unborn child. Fathers also felt more included in the pregnancy and childbirth process.

For Therapeutic Touch practitioners, these results were not surprising. Many nurses have taught Therapeutic Touch to relatives of sick patients, so that they could relieve pain for their family members when professional help was unavailable. These families report that their members become more sensitive to one another's feelings, and more aware of their own emotions. Communication improves, and relationships become more meaningful.

Therapeutic Touch has also been used successfully during labor and delivery. Dolores Krieger did not design her study to evaluate Therapeutic Touch during labor, and there exist no other studies that have done so. However, nurses who use Therapeutic Touch in the delivery room, and women whom they have treated during labor, report that it helps them to cope with the pain of their contractions. Therapeutic Touch does not necessarily decrease labor pain, as would pain medication, but it helps laboring women to relax. As the contractions become stronger and more frequent, some women report feeling exhausted and unable to continue. When they receive Therapeutic Touch, they find it easier to remain focused on the work of labor, and to avoid being overwhelmed by a feeling of panic that can come with the intense physical demand of each contraction. Laboring women have reported that Therapeutic Touch allows them to find an inner strength to contend with their labor. They also report that Therapeutic Touch quiets others in the room they are in, so there are fewer distractions.

Therapeutic Touch with Premature Babies

Since the 1970s, nurses have practiced Therapeutic Touch in the hospital nursery, as an adjunct to the medical care of premature infants. Physicians consider infants premature if they are born before the thirty-eighth week of the pregnancy. Some babies, born as early as the twenty-fourth week, are severely premature, have more difficulty surviving, and if they do, often have many health problems. Prematurity threatens survival because during the last three months of pregnancy, most of the body organs of the fetus are continuing to develop. The earlier the baby is born, the less some organs are able to function independently, and the greater the baby's physiological stress.

Premature babies differ from full term babies in many ways. They are less able to maintain their body temperatures. Premature infants do not have as much body fat as full term infants and so are not as well insulated against the cold. They have a higher ratio of surface area to weight that results in more heat loss to the environment. When they get cold, they must increase their metabolism to generate heat. They can become hypoglycemic and develop abnormalities in breathing, heart rate, and circulation.

Premature babies have problems in both the way their lungs function and in how their nervous system controls breathing.

Immature lungs do not stay inflated normally and are unable to transport oxygen into the bloodstream efficiently. The infant's immature nervous system does not regulate breathing in a normal fashion. Premature babies therefore have periods of apnea, where they stop breathing for a short time. As a result of these respiratory problems, premature infants often require mechanical ventilators to assist their breathing, and as a result are at risk for developing chronic lung disease. Premature babies are also at risk for the complication of pneumonia. Because their immune systems have not fully developed, they are more susceptible to infection.

Premature infants face a number of other risks, not all of which can be detailed here. These examples illustrate the fragility of their hold on life, and their need for constant medical and nursing care to ensure their survival. As the following case histories illustrate, Therapeutic Touch plays a role in treating many of these complications of prematurity.

Joanne O'Reilly is a nurse at a large hospital in the eastern United States. She has over seventeen years experience caring for premature infants in intensive care. For fifteen years, she has integrated Therapeutic Touch into the care of these babies. Most of her patients are fragile, weigh less than two pounds, and experience many of the complications of prematurity. She believes that Therapeutic Touch, when used with the usual highly sophisticated medical care that sick babies receive, makes a difference for premature infants.

One of her patients, Catherine, was born at the beginning of the seventh month of her mother's pregnancy, and weighed less than two pounds. Catherine suffered a pulmonary hemorrhage—bleeding into the lung—the day before she became Joanne's patient. After Joanne treated Catherine with Therapeutic Touch, the baby's condition stabilized. Catherine received daily Therapeutic Touch treatments, while her usual medical care continued. The baby progressed smoothly, had no setbacks, and was able to breathe without her respirator more quickly than most babies with the same problem. What was unusual about Catherine's progress was that the course of her recovery was so uncomplicated. She did not develop Respiratory Distress Syndrome (RDS), a more serious and chronic lung problem that often affects premature babies. Her nurses and doctors noted that the oxygen content of her blood improved after Therapeutic Touch. She ate well, and gained weight. Her family reported that on days that Catherine received Therapeutic Touch she was quiet and more able to rest.

Another of Joanne O'Reilly's patients was Laura, a baby who was born at the end of the sixth month of her mother's pregnancy, and weighed a little over one pound. Laura had many of the complications of prematurity and her physicians did not expect her to survive. She developed RDS and required a respirator for several months. She had abdominal surgery for necrotizing enterocolitis, an inflammation of the bowel sometimes occurring in preterm infants. She also lost her sight in one eye as a result of retinal detachment. This occurs in premature babies because of lack of sufficient blood supply to the retina, and because of changes that occur in the eye when the baby requires oxygen for a prolonged period. Laura underwent surgery on her other eye in an attempt to preserve her vision. Her prognosis was poor.

During Laura's eight months in intensive care, Joanne treated her frequently with Therapeutic Touch. Despite her complications, she recovered. Her eye surgery was successful, and the vision in one eye was preserved, despite her doctors' predictions of a poor surgical result. Laura's family was devoted to her, and her mother participated in her care. Joanne taught Laura's mother how to help with her baby's nursing care. She also taught Laura's mother how to center. Learning this first step of Therapeutic Touch helped both the mother and baby to remain calm, despite the medical complications.

Laura is now three years old. Although she is small—she

weighs eighteen pounds—she is learning and developing. Her sight remains in one eye. She has normal comprehension and use of language for her age and has far exceeded the expectations of her doctors and nurses.

For the babies mentioned here, and for many others who have received Therapeutic Touch, it is difficult to know the precise role that Therapeutic Touch has played in their recovery. In the opinion of the nurses caring for them, Therapeutic Touch seems to accelerate the healing process, and to soothe the babies so that they are more comfortable. Many of the parents of babies who have received Therapeutic Touch believe it has been instrumental in their children's recovery. Both the nurses and family members agree that it is the combination of highly sophisticated medical care with Therapeutic Touch that has been helpful, and that it is difficult to sort out the exact role that Therapeutic Touch plays.

Other nurses practicing Therapeutic Touch have had similar experiences to those of Joanne O'Reilly. Elly Leduc is a nurse at a large medical center in the Pacific Northwest. She has been a Therapeutic Touch practitioner since 1983, and has worked for many years caring for infants in a Level II nursery. Babies in Level II nurseries are not critically ill, but have a wide variety of medical problems, sometimes relating to complications of their delivery.

Elly reports using Therapeutic Touch to help babies with a variety of illnesses.[2] One of her earliest uses of Therapeutic Touch was in babies suffering from transient tachypnea. Excess fluid in the lungs after birth results in the baby's breathing becoming rapid and labored. Transient tachypnea typically resolves in twenty-four hours, and does not usually require medical treatment. Shortly after learning Therapeutic Touch, Elly treated one baby who was short of breath after birth. After treating the child for one or two minutes, Elly noticed that the baby's breathing slowed, she became comfortable and was able to rest. Because most cases of transient tachypnea resolve this quickly, a more serious problem, such as pneumonia, is often responsible if the baby's breathing does not slow in response to Therapeutic Touch.

Nurses using Therapeutic Touch are almost always able to calm irritable babies. Practitioners use it to soothe babies of smokers, and quiet babies with meningitis—an infection that causes inflammation of the lining of the brain. Some nurses who have treated babies of mothers addicted to cocaine report that Therapeutic Touch is one of the few things that can help these highly irritable babies.

Therapeutic Touch is also effective in treating babies and small children with chronic lung disease, one form of which—bronchopulmonary dysplasia (BPD)—affects babies who have had prolonged periods on respirators and have received oxygen for a long time, because of prematurity. Children with BPD have destruction of some of their lung tissue. As a result, they have less oxygen in their blood, and are also susceptible to lung infections. Elly Leduc has successfully used Therapeutic Touch in treating some children with BPD. Because there is actual damage to lung tissue, Therapeutic Touch will not reverse this, and the underlying problem remains. However, Leduc has discovered that children treated three times a week, over a period of at least two weeks, but optimally longer, experience fewer infections and have more energy. Their quality of life improves, despite the presence of the disease.

Leduc has instructed the parents of children with BPD in the steps of Therapeutic Touch, so that they can treat their own children at home. Because the treatment relieves anxiety for both the children and the parents, the families are better able to cope with the stresses of caring for a chronically ill child.

Most of what we know about Therapeutic Touch for infants comes from the clinical experience of its practitioners in hospital nurseries. In an attempt to evaluate its effects more scientifically, Rosalie Fedoruk, for her nursing doctoral dissertation, studied the effectiveness of Therapeutic Touch for reducing stress in premature infants.[3] The premature infant in intensive care is constantly stressed. Nurses and physicians handle some infants over one hundred times each day in the delivery of their routine care. Handling of premature infants can cause them to temporarily stop breathing, and can slow their heart rates. Dr. Fedoruk studied whether Therapeutic Touch could reduce the stress of handling associated with a routine nursing procedure—the taking of vital signs.

Researchers studied the effects of Therapeutic Touch on seventeen infants. Each infant received Therapeutic Touch on two occasions. The same babies received a mock Therapeutic Touch treatment on two occasions, in order to see if the effects of Therapeutic Touch would differ from those of simple human interaction. Researchers also compared the results of these treatments with the results of no treatment.

After a staff nurse had taken the infant's vital signs, a practitioner treated each baby with Therapeutic Touch, or the mock treatment, for about five minutes. After treatment, the babies rested for ten minutes. Observers then assessed the baby's stress level.

Dr. Fedoruk measured infant stress in two ways. Her first measure was a checklist of the babies' behavior called the Assessment of Premature Infant Behavior, which was developed by Harvard pediatrician T. Berry Brazelton. Together with his colleagues Als, Lester, and Tronick, he devised a way for an observer to assess patterns of an infant's behavior. By noting specific behaviors, an observer can tell if the baby is relatively stressed or relaxed. The most obvious indications of this are that a highly aroused baby will cry, and a very relaxed baby will sleep quietly.

The other measure of stress was the transcutaneous pressure of oxygen ($TcPO_2$) measured with a monitor attached to the baby's skin. $TcPO_2$ reflects both the oxygen content of the blood and the blood flow to the skin. Decreases in $TcPO_2$ sometimes occur when an infant is physiologically stressed.

Increases may occur when the baby is relaxed.

The study determined that infants receiving Therapeutic Touch were more relaxed when observers evaluated their behaviors according to the indicators on the checklist. There was no significant difference, however, between the groups in their $TcPO_2$.

Nevertheless, Dr. Fedoruk's study does demonstrate that Therapeutic Touch will decrease stress-induced behaviors in premature infants. The clinical experience of other nurses working in intensive care units with premature infants supports this finding. They report that Therapeutic Touch slows the baby's rate of breathing if it is too fast, and decreases rapid heart rate as the baby relaxes. They also note that infants in neonatal intensive care units who receive Therapeutic Touch have fewer feeding problems and gain weight faster. At present, this field would benefit from further studies to confirm both Dr. Fedoruk's findings and other nurses' independent observations. Despite the need for more research, the clinical experience with Therapeutic Touch in the premature nursery has been positive and virtually without risk to the infants.

Therapeutic Touch with Children

Older children also benefit from Therapeutic Touch. Linda Schill is a pediatric nurse who has practiced Therapeutic Touch for almost twenty years. For much of this time, she worked on a pediatric surgical unit at a large medical center in San Francisco, caring for seriously ill children after surgery. When she began to integrate Therapeutic Touch into their care, fellow staff members commented, "When you are working it's quieter here." She noticed that the children often responded to Therapeutic Touch by falling asleep afterwards. Some children were reluctant to receive Therapeutic Touch if they wanted to play or watch television, because they knew that the treatment would relax them too much to be active.

While working on the pediatric surgical unit, Linda noticed that children treated with Therapeutic Touch usually had their surgical wounds heal faster, and that their hospital stays were sometimes shorter than those of children who did not receive Therapeutic Touch. Other nurses who work with children in a variety of clinical settings share these observations. They also notice that the parents of children who receive Therapeutic Touch are often better able to cope with their child's illness. Linda often taught parents how to treat their children with Therapeutic Touch. She discovered that although it was very difficult for most parents to detach from the outcome of the treatment, they could learn to center and to balance their child's energy. This relaxed both the child and the parent, and allowed the parents to better participate in their child's care.

Besides playing a role in helping children get better, and assisting their parents to cope, Therapeutic Touch allows many children to die peacefully. One of Linda's patients was a four-year-old boy, Christopher, who was hospitalized after a bacterial infection spread to his bloodstream and caused endocarditis—an infection of his heart valves. Christopher became very ill, despite the best of medical care. His physicians eventually admitted him to the intensive care unit, where he had repeated seizures and cardiac arrests. The hospital staff resuscitated him many times, but he could not recover. Linda treated him with Therapeutic Touch during his illness. When it became apparent that he would not live, she helped his parents to accept that the doctors had done everything they could to help their child, but that he was dying. Christopher died peacefully, with his parents present. The staff who cared for him believed that his receiving Therapeutic Touch helped Christopher to die at peace, and helped his family to accept the inevitability of his death.

In 1980, Linda taught Therapeutic Touch and cared for

sick patients in a refugee camp in Thailand. The residents of the camp were Cambodians fleeing the atrocities of dictator Pol Pot. The camp housed both adults and children, many of whom were suffering from typhoid, tuberculosis, pneumonia, and malnutrition. Some refugees also experienced serious psychological problems as a result of seeing their families killed, or because of torture. At the refugee camp, which the United Nations sponsored, Linda taught Therapeutic Touch to the Cambodian hospital workers. Because Therapeutic Touch was effective in relieving pain and anxiety, the hospital staff felt that if they had to suddenly leave, the Cambodian hospital workers would be able to offer something to the other refugees. Because the Cambodians were accustomed to healing practices that were similar to Therapeutic Touch, they learned the technique very quickly, and treated patients effectively.

The staff at the refugee hospital noticed that children and adults who received Therapeutic Touch were calmer. Often Therapeutic Touch was the only method of pain relief available, because there was a shortage of medications. Due to Therapeutic Touch and other cross-cultural healing techniques native to the refugees, the cure rate in this hospital was higher than that of the other United Nations established hospitals in the area. As a result, the United Nations rewrote their protocol for treatment of refugees, using this more successful model to apply to their refugee work around the world. Although Therapeutic Touch may have played a role in the increased cure rate, the acceptance by the staff of the patients' cultural beliefs and customs also appeared to be an important factor in helping the patients to get better.

Although many Therapeutic Touch practitioners note that the technique is helpful in reducing fever in children, speeding the healing of fractures and wounds, and helping children to sleep, there have been few studies that examine the results of Therapeutic Touch scientifically. One study, published in

1990 by Nancy Kramer,[4] determined that Therapeutic Touch was effective in reducing the time needed to calm children after stressful experiences they experience as part of their hospital care.

This study evaluated the use of Therapeutic Touch in infants and young children from two weeks to two years, whom doctors had hospitalized for acute illness, surgery, or injury. Researchers studied thirty children. Half the children received Therapeutic Touch after a stressful experience—either blood drawing, an examination by the physician, or a surgical procedure. The remaining children received calming, casual touch after a similar stressful experience.

The researchers measured the children's pulse, skin temperature, and galvanic skin response to determine if the treatments were physiologically relaxing. They discovered that children receiving Therapeutic Touch relaxed more significantly, both three and six minutes after treatment, than did children receiving casual touch.

The clinical experience of both nurses and physicians is that Therapeutic Touch is effective in helping sick children in a wide variety of situations, when it is used in addition to their medical care. As we have seen, the practice of Therapeutic Touch enhances family relationships at the time of the birth of a newborn. It reduces pain and anxiety during labor and delivery. Therapeutic Touch helps premature infants to rest, gain weight, and reduces their physiological stress. Pediatric nurses have used it effectively to relieve pain and promote healing in older children and to help children to die peacefully.

Special Considerations in Working with Children

Therapeutic Touch relieves pain and induces relaxation for children more rapidly than for adults because children are often more open to the experience and more receptive to receiving help. Children also lack preconceived notions about their illness, or fixed ideas about sickness. The habitual patterns of thinking and feeling that partially affect the healing process in adults are not as prominent in children. As a result they often retain more healing energy during Therapeutic Touch than do adults.

Nurses who care for sick children generally treat them for short periods of time—generally only a few minutes. Small children, especially, have difficulty sitting still for longer treatments, and because children are rapidly responsive, prolonged treatments are usually not necessary.

The attitude and intent of the practitioner are always important during Therapeutic Touch, but they become more so when a child is the patient. Children are very aware of the emotional state of adults around them. If the practitioner becomes distressed by the child's pain, the child senses this and becomes even more upset. The practitioner needs to remain calm during the treatment, and not become overidentified with the child's feelings. This is especially important for nurses working with premature infants. Because suffering babies distress most people, nurses caring for sick infants can become emotionally drained easily. If the practitioner approaches the baby with empathy, but remains emotionally calm, she will be able to project this to the baby, who will quickly relax. If the practitioner is agitated because the infant is in pain, the baby senses this and becomes more fretful.

There are other special considerations to keep in mind when caring for premature babies. Because these infants have lost the protection of the intrauterine environment, they are often restless and irritable. Joanne O'Reilly, who has instructed other nurses in Therapeutic Touch techniques with premature babies, thinks of the baby as surrounded in a cocoon of blue. This mental image helps her to think of the baby as contained and soothed, as it would be if still inside its mother. As she gives Therapeutic Touch treatments, she thinks of the baby's energy as fluid and moving, like a stream of water. She balances the energy gently, slowing it down. If the energy feels fragmented—like static, or pins and needles—she thinks of it as smooth. Joanne recommends treating premature babies with Therapeutic Touch for only a few moments at a time. They are small and very responsive. If the practitioner treats them for too long a time, they can become irritable and uncomfortable.

The attitude of the parents also plays a role in promoting healing for sick children. It is understandable that parents may be fearful or anxious when a child is sick. If they feel the child's pain as their own, however, they run the risk of becoming overwhelmed by his difficulties, and then cannot help. If the parents remain calm, send loving thoughts to their child, and hope for the best, the sick child is better able to relax. While some parents have successfully treated their children using Therapeutic Touch, most find that it is difficult to detach from the need for a specific outcome of treatment. The normal investment of parents in a specific result, and their own anxiety about whether or not they can help, often interferes with treatment. Trained professionals are therefore often more effective.

Because healing is promoted when children have a creative outlet, parents can help by giving their children an opportunity to participate in life, in a way that is realistic given the limitations of their illness. If children can be active and involved with others, and busy with activities, they develop self-confidence. Despite the presence of illness, they can experience a part of themselves that is healthy and functioning.

7

Therapeutic Touch for Serious Illness

ALTHOUGH MODERN MEDICINE has made great strides in the twentieth century, there remain many diseases for which there is no reliable cure. Among these are AIDS, some cancers, and Alzheimer's disease. These illnesses inflict both physical and emotional suffering, and although long-term survival is possible, they are life-threatening. Patients burdened with any of these diseases face the long-term prospect of exacerbation and remission of illness, and an uncertainty of what the future will bring.

For the past twenty years, Therapeutic Touch practitioners have been treating cancer patients as an adjunct to their usual medical care. For the past ten years, both nurses and physicians have used Therapeutic Touch in the care of HIV positive individuals. More recently, some practitioners have treated older people with Alzheimer's disease. For each of these illnesses Therapeutic Touch appears effective in relieving symptoms associated with the disease, and in providing relief from emotional distress. Patients who receive Therapeutic Touch report that it enhances their feelings of well-being. Whether Therapeutic Touch plays a role in prolonging life is unclear. Some patients, as we shall see later in this chapter, believe that it has been instrumental in helping them to withstand the complications of their illness and has lengthened their survival. However, researchers have not studied this systematically. Almost all patients who receive Therapeutic Touch do so in addition to usual medical therapies for their illnesses. It is often difficult, therefore, to sort out which factors contribute to an increase in life span.

Therapeutic Touch for HIV Related Disease

HIV related illness first appeared in the United States in 1980, as an unknown disease affecting homosexual men in San Francisco and New York. In 1984, researchers identified the human immunodeficiency virus type I (HIV-1) as the causative agent of the disease. Since that time the disease has become pandemic. In the United States alone, just over 500,000 cases of AIDS were reported by the end of 1995. Scientists believe the AIDS virus has infected up to 2 million people in this country, most of whom are presently asymptomatic. About 18 million adults and 1.5 million children have been infected worldwide, most of these in Africa and Asia.

HIV-1 is transmitted through sexual contact and contaminated blood products. The latter was a risk in the United States from about 1978 until 1985, when blood banks implemented screening of transfused blood for the AIDS virus. HIV is also transmitted by injection with contaminated needles. This is a primary mode of transmission for intravenous drug abusers, and sometimes a risk in developing countries where health professionals reuse needles for injection without sterilization. The HIV virus is also sometimes transmitted perinatally. Mothers may infect their children before birth, at the time of delivery, or after birth through breast feeding.

In the United States, Australia, and Western Europe both

homosexual men and intravenous drug users are the major groups infected with HIV. However, heterosexual transmission is becoming more common. As a result of this trend, epidemiologists estimate that in the United States by the year 2000, up to 125,000 children under the age of eighteen will have lost their mothers to AIDS.[1] Although tragic, these facts should not be surprising. The predominant pattern of HIV transmission worldwide is heterosexual. In Africa, parts of Latin America, and the Caribbean, the ratio of infected males to females is 1:1, and transmission from mother to child is a major problem.

These statistics tell us that AIDS is a major public health problem worldwide, and one that is not going to disappear. It is a challenge to both our ability to organize effective systems of care for those affected, and to our human compassion.

The HIV virus attacks the cells of the immune system, eventually rendering them incapable of defending an infected person against a variety of other bacterial, fungal, and protozoal infections. Infected individuals suffer from pneumonia and gastrointestinal disturbances. Esophageal diseases, which cause pain and difficulty swallowing, are common. Chronic diarrhea, from both infectious and other causes, is also problematic. Patients with AIDS also may develop meningitis and brain abscess. They are more at risk for many kinds of cancer. The HIV virus results in a variety of complications that make this a difficult disease for physicians to treat, and causes physical, emotional, and mental distress for those who are infected.

Recent advances in medical care have helped to improve the length of survival for some HIV positive people. Most of the benefit has been the result of better treatments for the secondary infections that plague patients. Because of the ability of the HIV virus to develop resistance to drugs aimed against it, and because of its ability to change its structure, attempts to eradicate the virus itself with medication or prevent it with vaccines have so far been unsuccessful.

In our current efforts to treat the complications of AIDS and to provide emotional support to its sufferers, Therapeutic Touch has made a contribution. Nurses throughout the country, and some physicians, treat HIV positive people in hospitals and private practices. In a Therapeutic Touch treatment group in Seattle, the authors have treated many HIV positive patients over the course of their illnesses. As a result of this experience, we have learned that Therapeutic Touch helps to relieve pain, allay anxiety, and improve many of the difficult to manage symptoms of HIV positive people.

When they discover they are HIV positive, many people become fearful, and panic sometimes overwhelms them. Because AIDS is a disease that medicine cannot cure, patients become extremely apprehensive about what the future will hold. If they have had friends or relatives die of the disease, they anticipate that the worst of what they have seen will happen to them. At this stage, Therapeutic Touch helps by relaxing the patient, relieving the feelings of panic and helping him to adjust to the shock of the diagnosis.

After diagnosis, many people are well for up to several years without experiencing any complications. Therapeutic Touch can be useful at this stage because it helps recipients to maintain their energy. Perhaps even more important, it also helps them to identify with an inner self that is something more than their diagnosis. Jim Schultz is a long-term survivor who discovered he was HIV positive in 1985. Since shortly after his diagnosis, he has chosen to receive Therapeutic Touch in addition to his other medical care. He describes his experience and how Therapeutic Touch has affected him:

When I tested HIV positive in 1985, my doctor told me I had six to twelve months to live. When I heard this prediction, I started using cocaine more heavily. I decided if I had six to twelve months to live, I could probably kill myself in nine or ten months. When ten months went by and I was still here, I began to question my prognosis.

I returned to the doctor for repeat testing, thinking that maybe my test had been a false positive. Again, I tested HIV positive. My T cell count was 527, decreased from normal, but not yet dangerously low. Because of my cocaine abuse, my doctor pointed out that if I was trying to kill myself, I was doing a good job. It was right then that I realized that I wanted to live, not die.

After that visit to the doctor, I stopped using cocaine, stopped smoking, and stopped drinking any alcohol. I isolated myself from anyone or anything that could jeopardize my health. Because this was a very lonely time for me, I decided to get some support from a therapist who had worked with the Santa Cruz AIDS Project.

Besides being a therapist, Sally offered Therapeutic Touch as a part of her care. When she treated me with Therapeutic Touch, I could feel the energy move through my body. With my eyes closed I could feel where Sally was working. I could assist her. For example, I could visualize blue or green light coming in through my head, flowing down through my lungs and out my feet. As a result of being treated with Therapeutic Touch, I began to realize that I have control over how the energy flows through my body.

This sense of control also helped me understand that I could take some control over my illness. I could choose my response to what was happening, and make some decisions about my care. I became confident that I could help myself.

Therapeutic Touch has been part of a series of changes I have made that I believe contribute to my long-term survival. From the moment in the doctor's office that I decided I wanted to live I have done several things. I made an effort to find out what treatments were available. I made use of a network of people who were HIV positive, so that I could give and receive information about my illness and its care. I built up a regimen of things I could do for myself. I try to get enough physical rest, and I take dietary supplements. Emotionally, I don't buy into the gloom and doom that surrounds being HIV positive. I try to maintain a sense of humor. I know this is a life and death issue, but if I take it all too seriously I assure my demise. I have also tried to deal with emotional issues from the past and to resolve current problems with people as they arise. Mentally, I try not to run negative tapes. I don't dwell on my illness and the bad things that could happen. I also meditate on a regular basis.

Receiving Therapeutic Touch treatments helps me remain steady emotionally. When I get sidetracked and upset, it's usually at a time when I haven't received Therapeutic Touch for a while. Therapeutic Touch restores my balance. I don't know why this works, but confidence is a major part of what I get out of the treatments. I can do things now that I never could have done ten years ago. After a Therapeutic Touch treatment I feel complete and recharged. I have more energy to meet life's demands.

At the time this book goes to press, Jim Schultz has been HIV positive for over ten years, and remains free of any complications. He is not alone in being symptom free after many years of infection. Scientists are beginning to identify other long-term survivors, and major medical centers are studying them to determine what it is that makes them more the exception than the rule. Researchers believe that a less virulent strain of the HIV virus infects some people. Others have the ability to mount an immune response that better controls viral replication.

As noted in Chapter Five, scientists are beginning to demonstrate that our thoughts and feelings affect the level of immune cells in our blood. We are far from a complete understanding of how this fact translates into actual protection against disease. Nevertheless, it raises the possibility that a broad approach to treating HIV related illness, with attention to our physical, emotional, mental, and spiritual needs, may enhance our body's immunity and therefore its ability to contain infection. Therapeutic Touch is one modality that is part of this comprehensive approach. Its ability to induce the relaxation response suggests that it may enhance immunity. Even more important, the extra energy and confidence that its recipients report allow some people to live a creative and meaningful life, despite being HIV positive.

Although there are some long-term survivors who have integrated Therapeutic Touch into their care, there is no documented proof that it is responsible for increasing survival. Many Therapeutic Touch recipients have suffered serious complications secondary to their infection with HIV. For these patients, however, Therapeutic Touch plays a role in providing symptomatic relief, and sometimes speeds healing of certain infections.

One of the most common complications of infection with the HIV virus is Pneumocystis carinii pneumonia, commonly called PCP. PCP causes fever, cough, and shortness of breath. Treatment with Therapeutic Touch is effective both in slowing rapid respiration and relieving the cough associated with the pneumonia. When a practitioner treats a patient with pneumonia, she often detects congestion in the energy flow over the chest. Instead of the usual light flow of energy that feels like bubbling water, the practitioner feels a thick, sluggish sensation under her hands. She treats the patient by clearing this away, thinking of the energy as smoothly flowing and balanced. Sometimes after only a few moments of treatment, the patient's rapid breathing slows down, he feels more comfortable, and remains that way for several hours.

Relief of pain is another effect of Therapeutic Touch that benefits people suffering AIDS complications. Patients sometimes suffer chest pain secondary to pneumonia, headache caused by meningitis, or stomach and abdominal pain as a result of gastrointestinal infections. Clinical experience has demonstrated that Therapeutic Touch relieves pain in many of these situations, decreasing the patient's reliance on analgesic medication. One especially effective use of Therapeutic Touch is in the treatment of painful legs and feet that commonly bother many HIV positive patients. This condition, called peripheral neuropathy, is difficult to treat with medication. Therapeutic Touch is effective for lessening this pain, and sometimes relieving it completely. When the practitioner assesses the patient with peripheral neuropathy, she often finds that the energy flow to the legs is disrupted. Instead of feeling smooth under her hands, it feels dysrhythmic. To relieve the pain, the practitioner treats the whole patient, as described in Chapter Four, but also concentrates on balancing and smoothing the energy flowing down the legs. Because it is more difficult to relieve the pain of peripheral neuropathy than it is to treat other problems, the practitioner often needs to treat for a longer period of time, and to treat on a regular basis to see improvement.

Therapeutic Touch also plays a role in relieving some of the uncomfortable abdominal symptoms of HIV related illness. People with AIDS suffer from a variety of gastrointestinal problems, many of which cause abdominal pain and diarrhea. Therapeutic Touch can relieve this pain and sometimes can help diarrhea, depending on its cause. The practitioner should project a feeling of calm, and think of the patient's energy as slowing down and becoming more rhythmic and coordinated. Sometimes the practitioner and the patient can both make a mental image of a cobalt blue light bathing the abdominal area. This tends to slow down intestinal contractions and therefore relieve pain.

In the later stages of HIV infection many patients experience energy loss. Even if they have no bothersome symptoms, constant fatigue may disrupt their lives. The Therapeutic Touch practitioner can help these patients by giving short, frequent treatments. Because the lungs are vulnerable to infection in HIV positive patients, the practitioner, when treating, should direct energy through the chest. Recipients will also benefit from the practitioner's directing energy over the low back, where the adrenals are located, and over the solar plexus. After being treated this way, patients will often feel an increase in their overall energy that lasts for several days or longer.

Besides increasing the recipient's sense of vitality, Therapeutic Touch often helps them to feel more at peace. Sally Blumenthal-McGannon, who as a psychotherapist and Therapeutic Touch practitioner cares for many HIV positive people, describes its effects on some of her clients:

> One of the worst things about HIV is that it reinforces any feelings of low self-esteem that a person may have. Its sufferers sometimes feel tainted and contaminated. Therapeutic Touch helps because it triggers a place inside that allows a patient to feel good. The recipient begins to keep the illness separate from who they are. They *have* an illness, but they are not the illness.
>
> People who receive Therapeutic Touch often feel more peaceful. Life also takes on purpose and meaning. They often find a way to go out and make a contribution to others.
>
> I find, too, that clients who receive Therapeutic Touch often have more energy to make changes in their lives.

For example, some people who are HIV positive have become estranged from their families, who may disapprove of their lifestyle choices. I am impressed with how often Therapeutic Touch recipients make efforts to reconcile with their families, or mend other important relationships.

Sally's experience suggests that Therapeutic Touch plays a role in helping people with AIDS to resolve unfinished emotional issues. Despite physical discomfort, they feel more peaceful. If they get sicker, they approach death with a sense of calm, rather than fear and anxiety. One patient, who has been HIV positive since 1990, and suffered some of the complications of his infection, says:

Therapeutic Touch has helped me to maintain my overall health, and allowed me to feel better as a trend. I have a greater sense of well-being. I am a more positive person. I feel more peaceful and more at home inside myself.

The words of both patients and practitioners suggest that although Therapeutic Touch may not necessarily prolong life, it relieves suffering and enhances quality of life for HIV positive people. Therapeutic Touch promotes healing, not by preventing death, or even the progression of physical disease. Instead, it promotes a sense of inner peace and personal strength that allows the individual to continue to participate creatively in life, and to make some contribution to others in whatever way their physical limitations allow.

Therapeutic Touch and Cancer

Because of advances in therapy over the past twenty years, many cancers are now curable, especially if diagnosed in the early stages. Despite the ability of medical care to help many people, however, malignancies remain a leading cause of death. Therapeutic Touch plays a role as an adjunct to therapy for patients both in early stages of their illness, and later on for those patients whom medical therapies do not cure.

At the time of their diagnosis, many people with cancer experience profound anxiety. They are afraid of what the future may hold. If their physician has told them that their cancer is incurable, or made predictions about how much time they have to live, patients often become concerned about how much they can achieve in the short time they have remaining. Like patients when they first learn they are HIV positive, people who are told of a cancer diagnosis sometimes have feelings of disbelief, shock, and panic. However, unlike someone who is HIV positive, a person with cancer is aware that medical therapies can often cure their disease. Despite their concern, they are often hopeful. Therapeutic Touch helps at this stage by relieving the patient's anxiety so that he can make decisions about his care, and begin to adjust to the reality he must face.

At this early stage, the practitioner, when treating the patient, can help by doing the following:

—Think of the patient as being whole and in control. Although the cancer may be localized to a particular organ, do not focus on the tumor itself. Think of healing affecting the entire body.
—To decrease anxiety, send energy to the solar plexus and think of the patient as peaceful.
—Think of restoring order to the patient's body. Cancer is a disease of disorder: Malignant cells have lost the ability to grow in an organized way. The healing process involves restoration of the body's order.

As patients begin their treatment for cancer they may begin to experience uncomfortable symptoms related to their therapy. Some patients undergo surgery, and need to recover both from the effects of anesthesia, and from the surgery itself. When practitioners treat patients with Therapeutic Touch before surgery, they recover more quickly from anesthesia. When practitioners treat patients afterward, their surgical wounds heal faster.

Some patients receive drugs or radiation as part of their cancer therapy. Although these treatments can produce a variety of side effects, the most common are nausea, vomiting, and diarrhea. Therapeutic Touch is useful in relieving these specific side effects, and in decreasing the fatigue and lethargy that many patients experience when undergoing cancer treatments. Practitioners can help by doing the following:

—Treat the patient *before* he receives chemotherapy or radiation if possible. Experience has shown that early treatment reduces side effects.

—Continue to treat the patient on a regular basis. Cancer therapies often cause great fatigue. Regular treatment will increase his energy and will help relieve symptoms as they arise.

—Direct energy specifically over the area of the solar plexus to help reduce nausea and anxiety. The patient will feel better and have an overall sense of balance.

—While working over the solar plexus, direct energy over the liver. Work over the lymph nodes, as well. The liver and lymph nodes are often sites of cancer spread. Think of them as functioning in a healthy and orderly way.

From the patients' perspective, Therapeutic Touch increases their energy so that they can participate more fully in their usual activities. The treatments also often draw patients and their caretakers closer together. One patient,

Alicia, at age forty-eight, discovered she had colon cancer. She describes her experience:

> When I receive a Therapeutic Touch treatment, I have much more energy than I usually do. The treatment relaxes me, and keeps the chemotherapy from tiring me.
>
> When I receive Therapeutic Touch, I feel as if the practitioner approaches me as a whole person, not only as someone with a disease. I have a supportive human connection with another. Although my doctors are very good, I sometimes feel they segment my medical care. I have an oncologist, a surgeon, and an internist, each of whom approach part of the problem. With Therapeutic Touch, I have the feeling that the practitioner is treating all of me. I have an opportunity to form a different kind of relationship than the one I have with my physicians.
>
> Therapeutic Touch has been good for me. It has given me a new perspective, and helped me focus on what it takes to heal. For me, this has meant taking a broader approach to my treatment, and making some changes in my life.

Therapeutic Touch and Depression

Serious illness is often accompanied by depression. People with cancer, heart disease, AIDS, and multiple sclerosis, for example, are confronted with a future which they believe will cause deterioration in their physical abilities. They may be forced to make major life changes to cope with the demands of their illness, and they may fear the onset of pain. Sometimes, people with serious illness anticipate death and its losses. Chronic pain, for any reason, is often associated with depression. As already mentioned in Chapter Five, people with chronic pain cannot anticipate a future without discomfort. Their self-image becomes eroded because they are often unable to function physically in the way they would like.

Depression need not be secondary to physical illness. In fact, up to 20% of the general population suffers from depression. Regardless of the cause of the depression, there are certain things that depressed people share in common—low energy, low self-esteem, and feelings of hopelessness. Some people may be only mildly depressed. This form of depression is transient, usually triggered by some environmental stress, such as a problem at home or at work, and exists only for a period of days. Moderate and severe depression is longer-lasting and characterized by feelings of hopelessness that are not warranted by the situation the depressed person is experiencing. People who have more than mild depression often have a low self-image while they are depressed: They may feel worthless and guilty.

Depression is characterized by low energy. The depressed person often feels both physically and mentally fatigued. He may want to go for a walk, for example, but feels too tired to move. Because his energy is low, he cannot will himself into action. A depressed person is also self-absorbed. He becomes preoccupied with his problems. His thoughts and feelings of helplessness and hopelessness recur again and again. Because of his low energy, he often limits contact with others, which further reinforces his preoccupation with himself.

Anyone with more than mild, transient depression should seek medical care. There is effective therapy for depression which may vary depending on the cause, patient's age, and whether or not they have associated physical illness. The use of medication with or without psychotherapy provides relief for most people. Besides medical care, Therapeutic Touch can help in the treatment of depression. It is most useful, however, if it is used *early* in the development of the depression.[2]

The onset of depression is often heralded by a drop in a person's usual energy level. His everyday activities may begin to feel overwhelming. Because he feels tired, he begins to decrease contact with the outside world. If he is treated with Therapeutic Touch at this stage, his energy will increase. This makes it easier for him to mobilize his will to get better, and to be more active. Involvement in activity will boost his energy level and improve his self-confidence. This helps to counteract the self-absorbed negative thinking, which further lowers energy and undermines self-image.

Therapeutic Touch alone will not prevent the depression. It is critical that the depressed person wants to get better, and that he initiates some *action*, however small, to direct his energy outward. Physical excercise or spending time relating to others direct the depressed person's focus of energy away from himself. The patient's use of his will to get better and to *act* supports his system's intrinsic drive toward health.

When a Therapeutic Touch practitioner treats a depressed patient, the practitioner notices that the flow of energy under her hands feels sluggish. This reflects the fact that the depressed person's energy exchange with the environment is low. When the practitioner treats the patient, she should work gently, and rhythmically, while thinking of establishing balance to the energy flow. Because depression is often accompanied by anxiety and irritability, the practitioner should project feelings of calm support toward the depressed patient. This often alleviates the anxiety and relaxes the recipient.

Therapeutic Touch and Alzheimer's Disease

Alzheimer's disease is a gradual loss of intellectual capacity that usually afflicts the elderly, but may occur in younger people as well. Those who suffer from the disease experience degeneration and loss of nerve cells in the cerebral cortex, which causes the brain to atrophy. As a result, the person with Alzheimer's disease experiences deterioration of intellectual function called dementia.

Alzheimer's disease is usually a slowly progressive problem. Initially, patients may exhibit mild forgetfulness and an inability to perform up to their usual standards. They may also lose interest in their activities. In the middle stages of the illness, patients have more of an obvious inability to comprehend and to think clearly. The individual suffering from Alzheimer's disease may repeat the same actions or words over and over. His judgment becomes impaired. Because he is forgetful, he may begin tasks that he does not complete.

Although Alzheimer's disease represents primarily a deterioration in intellectual functioning, patients experience emotional problems as well. They may become depressed and apathetic. At other times they may be anxious and agitated, or act in odd and unpredictable ways. Patients are sometimes emotionally labile. They may fluctuate wildly in their emotions, appearing happy one moment and tearful the next.

In the late stages of Alzheimer's disease patients begin to deteriorate physically. They may stop eating and walking, become bedridden and die from pneumonia or other infections.

During the middle and later stages of the illness, patients present many challenges to the family members caring for them. The forgetfulness associated with the illness often places the patients in danger. They may wander from home and get lost, or they may begin tasks, such as cooking, which they forget to complete. The family members often find it difficult to cope with the emotional outbursts and agitated behaviors that the affected person exhibits. As a result, caretakers often eventually seek institutional placement for relatives with Alzheimer's disease.

Despite receiving the best of care, people who suffer from dementia often continue to exhibit agitated behavior. They may also have difficulty sleeping, partly because their confusion often worsens at night. Over the past several years, as the incidence of Alzheimer's disease has increased, some Therapeutic Touch practitioners have treated confused and agitated patients to see if their symptoms would improve. Lynn Woods, a geriatric nurse practitioner in Vancouver, has cared for elderly patients since 1975. Since 1985, she has worked as a nurse clinician and educator specializing in caring for elderly patients with psychiatric disorders, and patients with Alzheimer's disease. She describes her experience treating one patient:

Irene was a woman who was confused and disoriented. She often did not know where she was. She slept poorly at night, usually requiring sleep medication. She was unable to feed herself, and was often upset and agitated.

Irene lived in a long-term care facility, but one day she came to the hospital where I was working. To help her agitation, I treated her with Therapeutic Touch. After her treatment she began to smile appropriately and respond to humor. She seemed more present, more alert, and focused on her environment.

She returned to her residence. I received a call from the nurses there, telling me that she was now able to feed herself, and she had not required any sleep medication. As a result of this experience, the staff at the long-term care facility requested that I teach Therapeutic Touch to them. They then were able to treat Irene on a regular basis, and offer treatment to their other patients as well.

The nurses found that patients receiving Therapeutic Touch were calmer and suffered less emotional distress. They had more of an awareness of their surroundings, and sometimes could be more independent in their care.

As a result of her experience, Lynn decided to examine scientifically the ability of Therapeutic Touch to affect agitation in patients with Alzheimer's disease. While at the University of Washington, she studied fifty-seven patients from three long-term care facilities. Lynn divided the patients into three groups. Nurses treated one group with Therapeutic Touch, and another group with a mimic treatment. A third group had no change in their care. Before the groups received their treatments, impartial observers, who knew nothing about the experiment, monitored the patients' behavior for three days. The observers used a list of specific behaviors, called the Agitated Behavior Rating Scale, to measure the frequency and intensity of agitated behaviors. This scale, developed by D. L. Bliwise and colleagues, was adapted by the researchers specifically for use with Alzheimer's patients. The observers noted the frequency and intensity of specific behaviors exhibited by the patient. These included searching and wandering, tapping and banging, pacing, and vocalization. This last behavior is characterized by repeating the same thing over and over, regardless of the response given by caretakers.

The observers rated the intensity and frequency of the behaviors every twenty minutes, for ten hours a day, for days one, two, and three of the experiment. On days four, five, and six, the patients received either Therapeutic Touch, the mimic treatment, or no treatment. The practitioners treated each patient twice daily. On days seven, eight, and nine, the researchers gave no treatments, but once again the observers rated the agitated behaviors of the patients, to see if the treatments had made any difference.

The researchers discovered that patients receiving Therapeutic Touch had a significant decrease in disruptive behaviors compared to patients receiving no treatment. They also had fewer disruptive behaviors than the patients receiving the mimic treatment, but these results were not statistically significant. The researchers also noted that the agitated behaviors of the patients who had received Therapeutic Touch decreased incrementally each day they were observed after treatment. That is, there were fewer agitated behaviors on day three after treatment than there were on day two, and fewer on day two than day one. This suggests that the effects of Therapeutic Touch somehow amplified with the passage of time.

Lynn Woods' experiment provides scientific verification of her clinical observation that Therapeutic Touch affects the agitated behaviors of Alzheimer's patients. Because the mimic treatment also decreased agitated behaviors somewhat, we need additional research to sort out the contribution of human contact alone to the change in patient behavior. Despite this, Therapeutic Touch clearly does decrease the patients' agitated behaviors, and does so without risk of harm. When disruptive behaviors decrease, nurses are better able to provide care, and the environment becomes more peaceful for all patients and staff. Therapeutic Touch in this way plays a useful role as an adjunct to care for the fragile elderly who suffer from dementia.

The experience of patients with Alzheimer's disease, HIV related illness, and cancer suggests that Therapeutic Touch often relieves some of their suffering and improves the quality of their lives. It makes a major contribution to the well-being of many people who face life-threatening illness. Therapeutic Touch does not hold out the promise of cure of any one of these conditions, but its ability to relieve pain, reduce anxiety, and alleviate some of the symptoms of illness makes it a valuable adjunct to care for the seriously ill.

Therapeutic Touch for the Dying

EIGHTY PERCENT OF Americans die in the hospital. This trend has been increasing since the 1940s, and marks a departure from the custom of dying at home, which was the rule until the early part of this century. To some extent, the increase in our dying in the hospital has paralleled the development of medical technology. Patients seek hospital care for the promise of relief or recovery that was not available until more recently. Advances in the treatment of cancer, for example, mean that patients receive chemotherapy and radiation treatments in addition to surgery. Because there is usually some treatment that can be offered, cancer patients have more hospital admissions than they did forty or fifty years ago, and they are more likely to die in the hospital than at home.

Cardiac patients, as well, are hospitalized more than in the past. Advances in medication and hemodynamic monitoring in intensive care units mean that there are more therapeutic options in treating both atherosclerotic heart disease and heart failure. Patients with serious heart disease are likely to be hospitalized for treatments that may prolong their lives, even for a short time. Cardiac patients who died at home in the earlier part of the century now die in the hospital while trying new therapy, or because those treatments have failed.

Health professionals view death differently now than they did in the past before medicine was so technological. Many physicians and nurses consider death to be a failure of their therapies, instead of a natural inevitable process. Because so much more *can* be done, some physicians and hospital ethics committees often decide that it *should* be done, even when life may be extended only days or weeks. When dying patients can no longer be helped medically, they are often isolated in rooms far from the nurses' station. They are sometimes avoided by the overworked staff, who spend more time attending to the patients who will survive their hospital stays. Patients dying in intensive care units, on the other hand, are well-attended by competent and usually caring staff, but often separated from friends and families at a time when their presence is the most important.

As in-hospital death has become more common, we have become insulated from the dying process. In the early 1900s children experienced the deaths of their grandparents, and sometimes their parents and siblings, as natural events that occurred at home. The dying people were not separated from their families, and the survivors experienced death as part of the life cycle. More recently, as death has been relegated to the hospital, many of us have never witnessed the death of a family member, and feel uneasy in its presence. Death has become invisible. It is something that happens away from the rest of us, who are busy living. As a result, the dying are sometimes isolated from those closest to them at a time when their greatest need is to understand the significance of their relationships and to resolve any remaining difficulties with others.

There are growing signs, however, that some of our attitudes toward death are changing. Over the past twenty-five years, the hospice movement has educated us to the importance of the patient's need to die as free from pain as possible, with attention to his emotional and spiritual needs, as well as his physical ones. The availability of home hospice care has allowed many people to remain at home while dying, instead of dying in the hospital. Physicians also have become more uncomfortable prolonging life for the terminally ill. In a survey published in 1993 by M. Z. Solomon and his colleagues, many physicians expressed concern that they were overtreating their dying patients.[1] The researchers questioned 687 physicians and 759 nurses in five hospitals. Seventy percent of the resident physicians and 47% of all respondents responded that they had violated their conscience when providing care to the dying. Seventy-five percent of this group felt that overly zealous treatment, not undertreatment, was their main concern. Many physicians believed that patients were resuscitated too aggressively. Seventy-eight percent of the resident physicians and 60% of the medical attendings admitted to being sometimes or almost always concerned that patients were placed on mechanical ventilators inappropriately. An even higher number—83% of residents and 61% of medical attendings—expressed concern about the overuse of cardiopulmonary resuscitation.

In another recent survey,[2] family physicians agreed that communication between doctor and patient was the most effective tool in helping patients to die. The doctors believed that the sharing of their feelings with their patients and family members helped them to better understand and care for the dying. This survey reflects the belief that care of the terminally ill requires more than medical technology, and more than concern on the part of the physician. Assisting patients who are close to death requires that physicians and nurses possess communication skills and an understanding of their own emotional state and that of their patient. As many experts on the care of the dying have pointed out, it is the gift of the human presence of the caretaker that is most significant to the dying person. The dying patient often feels fearful and vulnerable. If he can rely on a relationship that will continue, regardless of the uncertainties he will face, he can approach death knowing that he will not be abandoned.

During the past twenty years, many nurses and physicians have integrated Therapeutic Touch into the care of the terminally ill in hospitals, hospices, and at home. Therapeutic Touch quiets both the practitioner and patient, and makes them more aware of each other's feelings. It fosters communication and comforts the dying with another human presence. Even more significantly, when the trained practitioner conveys a sense of peace to the dying person, the patient experiences relief of anxiety, some relief of pain, and often dies more peacefully. The practitioner, as well, is often profoundly affected by assisting the dying process.

Clinical Experience with Therapeutic Touch

George Clark is a registered nurse who has worked for the past ten years at an extended care facility in Oregon. He received his RN degree at the age of seventy-one, and shortly afterwards became a nursing supervisor. George was born in New York City, attended high school there, and in 1937 he joined the Navy. After discharge from the Navy, he joined the Air Force when the Japanese bombed Pearl Harbor. He was the navigator of an Air Force B-29, and flew thirty-five missions over the Pacific during World War II. After the war, George returned to New York and worked for over thirty years as an engineer for the Long Island Railroad. During his last eleven years with the railroad he was the head of the Brotherhood of Locomotive Engineers.

After retiring from the railroad, George earned a bachelor of arts in liberal studies, then attended nursing school. Just prior to graduation he learned Therapeutic Touch, a course offered as an elective part of his nursing school curriculum.

In the 290-bed extended care facility at which George works, one third of the residents are living in a residential setting, and are able, with some assistance, to meet their own everyday needs. The remainder of the patients need more nursing care. Although some of the patients are expected to recover and go home, the majority have chronic medical conditions with which their families are unable to cope. Many of the patients are elderly.

In describing his experience using Therapeutic Touch with patients, George says:

> My philosophy is that when the elderly come to a nursing home or extended care facility they have been through some pretty traumatic times. The decision to put a parent into a nursing home is one that is very painful for the people who are burdened with making that decision. The residents themselves face the prospect of loss of control, as well as the realization that they are a lot closer to the end of life than the beginning. Most of my patients have illnesses so advanced that any so-called cure is just about out of the question. My belief in working with my elderly patients is that we owe them, at the very least, a peaceful and dignified death.
>
> As nursing supervisor, I have the opportunity of keeping track of the conditions of patients in the whole facility. I know which patients are facing death, and I make a point of visiting them every shift, at least. The first thing I do when treating dying patients is to balance their energy. Passing my hands around their heads brings such a dramatic change, it's really amazing. I see right before my eyes, in just one or two passes, peace, relaxation, and an ease to the labor of breathing. It's very obvious and very satisfying to me to be able to bring this help to people who are dying.
>
> As I balance the energy, I think to myself that the

energy is being presented to the patient for the best use that the body is able to put to it. If the patient has pain or difficulty breathing, I work more specifically over the affected areas.

Almost inevitably, after the administration of Therapeutic Touch, the patient becomes calmer. I know that they pass through the dying process in a less stressful way. As I treat them, I tell them they need not be afraid. It is not unusual that within twelve to eighteen hours after receiving Therapeutic Touch, the patient dies. I don't claim that Therapeutic Touch hastens their death, or changes the length of time they are going to survive. I am convinced, though, that it helps them in the passage.

The practice of Therapeutic Touch has changed the way I live. It's changed the things I think about and the things of which I am aware. I dedicate my time, hopefully, to helping someone else along the road, not only at the time of their death, but at all times—whether it's someone I meet in the course of my work, someone I meet in the street, or someone I've known for years. It is impossible to go through Therapeutic Touch training and begin to practice without being changed in a fundamental way.

Like George Clark, Dr. Gary Bachman has several years of experience in treating dying patients with Therapeutic Touch. Gary is a naturopathic physician in Mt. Vernon, Washington. Before studying naturopathic medicine at Bastyr University, he was a registered nurse. From 1979 to 1990, he cared for oncology patients, both at St. Peter's Hospital in Olympia and Providence Hospital in Seattle. Some of Gary's patients were admitted to the hospital for curative chemotherapy. Others, more seriously ill, were hospitalized for therapies to relieve uncomfortable symptoms, or because family members were unable to care for them at home.

Before learning Therapeutic Touch, Gary felt that his professional training had not prepared him to ease the mental and emotional distress of his dying patients. Although he provided regular nursing care, and administered medical therapies, he noticed that these measures could do only so much for people who were sometimes hopelessly ill. He saw his patients suffer in silence because they felt guilty complaining about treatments which might be uncomfortable but held out the promise of cure. Although some patients had the emotional support of their families, or of the hospital chaplain, many did not have anyone on whom to rely.

At the time he was feeling a need to offer something more to his patients, he cared for a dying cancer patient who taught him the power of the human presence in helping the dying. He describes this experience:

Carol was a woman who had multiple myeloma—a kind of cancer that is associated with destruction of the bone marrow. Because of the involvement of her bones, she was in constant pain everywhere. The night was a difficult time for her because she was unable to sleep, and always uncomfortable.

One night while I was working, Carol was continually restless. Her room was close to the nurses' station, where we could watch her closely. I was in and out several times, helping her to change position, and giving her pain medication, which didn't seem to be making any difference. I realized there was nothing else I could do. I had been coming in and out of the room, without staying very long. This time, instead of leaving, I sat and held her hand. Within about thirty seconds she calmed down. Her breathing became relaxed. A sense of peace filled the room. I stayed for five or ten minutes, and then left to care for other patients. Each time I passed her room I looked inside. She remained peaceful for the next two hours. The next time I checked on her she had died quietly.

I felt that I had been a contributor to her peaceful death, not by anything I was trying to do to help, but simply be being with her. My human presence was more supportive than all of my other efforts to help.

Shortly after caring for Carol, Gary learned Therapeutic Touch. He experienced this as an intentional way of using his presence to help his patients. Like other practitioners, by projecting feelings of quiet and calm toward the dying patient, he is able to help the sick person relax, and reduce his pain. Since learning Therapeutic Touch over twelve years ago, he has treated hundreds of dying cancer patients. From his perspective, Therapeutic Touch makes a significant difference for most people who are dying. Therapeutic Touch can calm agitated patients, and helps them to accept death when it is inevitable. The dying person's acceptance often makes it easier for the family to give their loved one permission to go—something that often brings peace of mind to the dying person. Gary describes one patient he treated:

David was a young man with advanced testicular carcinoma. After he was admitted to the hospital, the medical staff started administration of intravenous morphine, to control his pain and help with his restlessness and agitation. At first the medication was helpful, and then his restlessness returned. His physician ordered him another medication, which was ineffective.

After we had done what was medically possible, I treated David with Therapeutic Touch. I thought of him as peaceful and relaxed. He became calm and his breathing rate slowed. We decreased his morphine drip, and finally were able to stop it. I taught his family members how to do Therapeutic Touch, and they treated him intermittently. David remained pain-free and breathed comfortably, off morphine, until he died peacefully several days later, with his family's support.

In addition to helping the patient, Therapeutic Touch prevents the nurses who use it from becoming exhausted by working for long periods of time with very sick patients. Because dying patients and their families experience so much grief, and their needs for support are constant, nurses and physicians who work with them sometimes experience what is commonly called "burnout"—a chronic exhaustion which keeps them from being able to meet the needs of their patients as well as they would like.

When a practitioner uses Therapeutic Touch, she centers herself and projects thoughts of peace to the dying patient. Because the practitioner is calm, she is a source of stability and support to the dying person. When her own emotions are quiet, the practitioner is less likely to be upset by the painful feelings of the patient and family members. Centering helps the practitioner to avoid becoming emotionally drained. Sally Blumenthal-McGannon, a psychotherapist and Therapeutic Touch practitioner in California, describes how centering helps her to be effective in her care of dying patients:

Before becoming a therapist I worked as a hospital nurse; then almost twenty years ago, I discovered Therapeutic Touch and became a hospice nurse. The process of learning the technique, including the capacity to center myself, enhanced my ability to function as a nurse. As a hospital nurse, death had been the enemy—it represented a failure every time a patient died. Now, the more Therapeutic Touch I provided to my hospice patients, and sometimes to their family members, the more calm and peace prevailed, as I realized I too had become more peaceful with death.

I once cared for Joy, a woman who was dying from

cancer. She experienced a great deal of abdominal pain. She was also so frightened of dying, she was afraid to go to sleep at night. Each night I stayed with her I would do Therapeutic Touch, focusing on the pain in her abdomen. Not being attached to the results, one of the keys to effective Therapeutic Touch, I would work on Joy's abdomen, and let it go. One morning when she awoke she said, "Oh no." I asked her what was wrong and she told me she didn't want to wake up. She was in such a wonderful place, she didn't want to come back. I smiled, said good-bye and started to drive home when what she said hit me. I drove back and asked her again about what had happened. She thanked me for helping her get to a more peaceful place. I realized then that even though I had worked on the pain in her abdomen, that because I was centered and projected peaceful thoughts, she had become calm, moving to a place that felt safe to her. Not being attached to results, just doing my best and letting it go, allowed Joy to move into a peaceful place. She died quietly a few days later.

Besides helping to relieve the fear of dying patients, Therapeutic Touch plays a role in comforting the families and friends of the dying. Many practitioners have taught Therapeutic Touch to family members who have expressed an interest in learning. Gary Bachman has involved many cancer patients' relatives in their care. He believes that as patients become sicker and closer to death, the people who are close to them shift from playing an active role helping them to get better, to a passive role—waiting for death. They are afraid of their impending loss, and have no idea how to comfort or console the dying person. Therapeutic Touch allows family members to take an active role in caring for the dying and gives them a way to relate to the dying person which doesn't involve talking. Gary and other practitioners have encouraged children to be present when a dying relative is receiving Therapeutic Touch. The family is encouraged to be together, and children are a part of the process that brings peace to the dying person.

Dying people have an overwhelming need to resolve difficulties in their relationships with loved ones. Therapeutic Touch often sets the stage for this to occur. By providing a nonverbal way for people to express their caring, it promotes healing in the relationships of family members. Often the gentle projection of affection and peace toward the dying person is more powerful than words in communicating the feelings of family members.

Before attending nursing school, Sandra Revesz worked for several years as a licensed massage therapist and Therapeutic Touch practitioner. As a student nurse she cared for several patients with AIDS:

In 1987, I was a second-year nursing student at the University of Washington. We had just started seeing people with AIDS in the hospitals in Seattle, and we were still learning how best to care for them. The patients were placed in rooms with big signs outlining the precautions the staff needed to take upon entering. At that time, these included wearing gowns, gloves, and masks.

Because of the time involved in dressing in protective gear to go into the rooms, the patients' contact with nurses was limited to procedures and medication administration. There was little time to provide emotional support, or other extras. Each of the patients felt extremely isolated and alone.

One day I came into work and the nurses said, "There's a young man in there dying, and his mother is terribly distressed. She won't sleep or leave the room or even eat." I walked into the room thinking I'd offer massage to settle things down.

A very tall young man lay in bed, quite emaciated, receiving an intravenous morphine infusion. His mother was leaning over the bed, obviously exhausted. Only the week before, this young man had called home to Kansas to let his mother know he was dying of AIDS. His father, brother, and sister had not been able to call or speak with him, but his mother had come.

He desperately needed some rest, but as long as his mother stayed right by his bed, neither of them was going to get much sleep. I went to the end of the bed, introduced myself, and suggested that I do Therapeutic Touch. His mother said anxiously, "Do anything that will help!" As I started my Therapeutic Touch treatment, he leaned up and whispered to me, "I don't need this, *she does*." He was right. So, after a few moments I went to her shoulders and began rubbing them from behind. I asked him then to describe his favorite place, where he felt most relaxed.

He thought for a minute, then said, "The beach, on the northwest point of the Olympic Peninsula. I love to run on the beach barefoot with the wind in my hair. I love the sound of the waves crashing, and the seagulls crying. I love to breathe the salt air in and run for miles."

His mother was not relaxing at all. If anything, her shoulders were tighter. She couldn't relax watching her sick child, so I suggested she look out the window at a patch of blue sky. I began to work on her shoulders, and then slowly began to balance the energy over her back and legs. I asked her to tell us her favorite place. She said, "Oh, right here with my son." He said, "No, Mom, somewhere else, where you were relaxed." "Well," she said, "not the ocean. I can't swim and I hate the water. Just tell me again about your place." He began to repeat, "The sun on my face, the wind in my hair, running in bare feet on wet sand . . ."

And then she said, "Fields of wheat. When I was a young girl, I would run to the top of a hill and lie down in the tall golden wheat and watch the waves it made. I loved the feel of the sun on my face, and the sound of the birds overhead."

Her shoulders relaxed and the feeling in the room changed completely. I kept my hands gently moving, continuing Therapeutic Touch, as the two of them went on this trip together, sharing their places of joy and peace. When I left they were more relaxed, and something had changed between them.

The nurses told me that shortly after I left he fell asleep for hours, and she left the room for the first time in two days, to get something to eat. He died the next day. I knew for them there would be so much left unsaid, but they had had that moment together.

Special Considerations in Using Therapeutic Touch with the Dying

Birth, life, and death are a universal pattern. All living things, from the smallest one-celled organism to the largest star, will die. We, too, are part of this natural life cycle. From the point of view of most Therapeutic Touch practitioners, death represents a transition from one kind of existence to another. Although death marks the end of our physical existence, our consciousness continues. From this perspective, our sense of awareness, and our ability to register our experience, survives death. The belief in death as a natural process of transition from one form of existence to another leads to a calm acceptance of its inevitability for us all. The idea that consciousness continues implies that our relationships with loved ones can continue in some form after death. Dying people who believe they will continue to exist approach death with less anxiety than do those who fear oblivion. Family members who assume that a link with their loved one can continue do not feel as desolate at the loss of their physical presence.

Not all people share the conviction that consciousness continues after death. Nevertheless, Therapeutic Touch can help most people who are dying by creating a peaceful and calm atmosphere. This will help them to approach death with less anxiety and therefore less physical pain, as well. If the family can send thoughts of love and goodwill to the dying person, the transition becomes easier. Although the dying person is leaving the physical body and may be too weak to communicate verbally, he can respond to the thoughts and feelings of others.

Therapeutic Touch practitioners and family members can assist the dying if they keep certain things in mind.

—The dying person is an open energy system. As he comes closer to death, he becomes more sensitive to his environment. He may be easily irritated by loud noise or harsh lights. He may sense the feelings of caretakers and family more acutely than before, especially if they are anxious and distressed. When treating the patient with Therapeutic Touch, the practitioner thinks specifically of quieting the patient's energy and harmonizing its flow. This helps him to relax. A dying person will absorb energy very slowly, and therefore needs slow, gentle treatment.

—The dying person's energy is often very low. Constant physical pain is tiring, and in addition, patients often have many emotional issues to resolve. Both grief at saying good-bye to friends and family, and the need to resolve remaining issues in their relationships, demand energy. As a result, the dying person becomes fatigued and sometimes feels scattered. After receiving Therapeutic Touch, many dying people report that they are more in touch with their inner self and are not affected as much by their physical distress.

—When working with the dying, the Therapeutic Touch practitioner needs to remain centered, so that she can treat effectively without being overwhelmed by the emotions of the patient and family. The practitioner can then be a source of stability and strength and can help others tolerate their painful feelings.

—While treating the dying person, the Therapeutic Touch practitioner can silently convey to him that he has permission to go. Sometimes the sick person lingers because he is aware his death will grieve his loved ones. He may feel guilty, or simply wish to spare them pain. If the practitioner silently conveys an acceptance of the impending death, the dying person often feels released, and the family is more able to accept the inevitable.

—The sense of touch is a powerful way of maintaining contact with a dying person, who may be too weak to speak, and unable to see. Some practitioners hold the patient's hand, while working gently over the area of the heart. At the same time they send thoughts of peace to the dying person, and think of him as whole. The patient generally experiences a profound sense of peace.

For the dying person, healing is not the curing of his physical disease. Instead, the transformation that occurs at death is part of the healing process. Therapeutic Touch for the dying does not restore the body to health, but aids the dying transition. Although it plays a different role than in situations where physical recovery is possible, many of its previously described effects are the same. Therapeutic Touch eases pain for the dying person. It calms him and reduces fear. Therapeutic Touch sometimes helps the dying person feel more connected to family and loved ones and to resolve remaining difficulties with them. Perhaps most important, Therapeutic Touch restores an inner order, which contributes to the dying person's emotional and mental strength and fosters peace of mind.

9

❧❧

Horizons

Since originating Therapeutic Touch, both Dolores Krieger and Dora Kunz have taught the technique to thousands
of nurses and other health professionals. Their pupils have,
in turn, taught Therapeutic Touch in hospitals, colleges, and
schools of nursing throughout the United States and Canada.
For the past twenty years, workshops for Therapeutic Touch
practitioners have taken place annually, both at the Orcas
Island Foundation in the Pacific Northwest and at Pumpkin
Hollow Farm in upstate New York. These workshops in-
struct about two hundred health professionals each year in
each location. Nurses, physicians, and psychotherapists attend these workshops, and then return home to integrate
Therapeutic Touch into their practices, teach others the technique, and research its effectiveness.

In North America, there are two membership organizations for Therapeutic Touch practitioners. In the United
States, the Nurse Healers Professional Associates serves as an
information network for its members and a source of referrals for individuals interested in locating Therapeutic Touch
practitioners or teachers. Membership in the Nurse Healers
Professional Associates is open to nurses and other health

professionals. The organization's purpose is to educate its members in Therapeutic Touch and other healing modalities, and to develop knowledge about the effectiveness of the techniques.

In Canada, both Ontario and Alberta provinces have organizations called The Therapeutic Touch Network. The membership and purpose of these networks is similar to that of Nurse Healers Professional Associates. The Therapeutic Touch Network can help individuals locate practitioners throughout Canada. The Network can also provide referrals for groups or organizations seeking Therapeutic Touch teachers. Recently, they have established guidelines for Therapeutic Touch practitioners who would like to become teachers for other health professionals. They suggest that teachers of Therapeutic Touch have at least three years of experience, have studied with at least three practitioners, and mentored with another teacher before teaching independently. Although it is difficult to establish guidelines to assess the skill of a Therapeutic Touch practitioner or teacher, the Therapeutic Touch Network's suggestions ensure that teachers they recommend have had enough experience as practitioners to become skilled, and have had the opportunity to treat a wide variety of problems.

Dora Kunz and Dolores Krieger originally designed Therapeutic Touch to be incorporated into nursing practice. They conceived of it as an extension of care that nurses provide to sick patients, both in the hospital and in outpatient settings. As other health professionals have learned Therapeutic Touch and recognized its benefits, they have adapted it for use in their fields. Some psychologists, for example, use Therapeutic Touch at the beginning or end of counseling sessions. They find that clients treated at the beginning of the session often feel more connected to the therapist and talk more openly about their difficulties. Clients treated at the end leave the session relaxed and feeling more confident. Licensed massage therapists, as well, incorporate Therapeutic Touch into their massage techniques. Massage therapists often treat muscular injury and orthopedic injury. Massage promotes healing of specific injury by speeding circulation to and from the affected area. When therapists use massage for treatment of specific injury, they tend to concentrate on the affected body part. When Therapeutic Touch is added as a component of massage, the therapist focuses not on the specific injury alone, but on the integrated working together of the body. Besides speeding the resolution of a specific injury, massage combined with Therapeutic Touch promotes relaxation and stress reduction.

Although some physicians have been trained in Therapeutic Touch, it is often difficult for them to use the complete technique in their practices because of the pressure of seeing large numbers of patients in a limited time. Health professionals who cannot give complete treatments, however, often incorporate some of the steps of Therapeutic Touch as they see their patients. Busy physicians and nurses center themselves before seeing each patient, make a clear intent to help, and project thoughts of peace and calm toward each person. These things seem deceptively simple, but can be very effective. Practitioners who use these principles of Therapeutic Touch, even if they cannot treat the patients completely, report that they can see large numbers of patients without becoming physically and emotionally exhausted. Even more important, practitioners feel there is always something they can offer their patients. In cases where all of their available therapies have been ineffective, this is especially helpful. Physicians and nurses who use Therapeutic Touch feel more connected to their patients as people, and find their work more rewarding.

Patients, as well, benefit from having access to both modalities—their usual medical care plus Therapeutic Touch. As we have seen earlier, Therapeutic Touch can decrease their pain and anxiety and promote the healing process. It improves their sense of well-being and adds to their quality of life.

As mentioned in earlier chapters, both the originators of Therapeutic Touch and its many practitioners view its practice as an adjunct to traditional medical care, not a replacement. For this reason, health professionals are the most appropriate practitioners of Therapeutic Touch. They are trained to understand the complexities involved in caring for the sick, and they approach patient care in a scientific manner.

Some practitioners, however, who have taught Therapeutic Touch to family members of the sick believe that it plays a role in improving relationships within the family and should be taught to those interested and motivated to learn. As mentioned in Chapter Five, Dolores Krieger's study of the effect of husbands treating their pregnant wives with Therapeutic Touch demonstrated that it improved marital satisfaction for the couples who used the technique before childbirth. In an effort to add to our understanding of its effects on family relationships, Dr. Patricia Winstead-Fry is currently teaching Therapeutic Touch to the caregivers of cancer patients. She will measure whether Therapeutic Touch will improve quality of life for the patients, and reduce the emotional and mental burden of the caregivers.

There are specific situations where having a family member trained to do Therapeutic Touch can be useful. Many patients with serious diseases, people who are dying, and those in chronic pain often do not have access to health care professionals on a daily basis. Relatives who can center, project feelings of calm, and gently balance the patient's energy field can often help the patient relax, decrease his pain, and promote sleep. The difficulty that sometimes emerges for family members in treating a sick relative is that very often the patient communicates his anxiety in verbal and nonverbal ways to the relative trying to help. The family member becomes ineffective because he feels the patient's anxiety and makes it his own. He is therefore unable to project calm and peaceful thoughts. With training and practice, however, motivated people can learn to temporarily put aside their own feelings of anxiety and project calm.

Dr. Krieger's study, in fact, suggests that Therapeutic Touch can be practiced successfully by those who are not health professionals if they have been instructed and supervised in using the technique. The skilled use of Therapeutic Touch, however, requires practice and dedication to develop. For this reason, most advanced practitioners of Therapeutic Touch are health professionals, whose lifelong interest is in how best to help the sick. Nurses and physicians are trained to remain calm when patients are anxious and distressed. Most who practice Therapeutic Touch meditate on a daily basis. This routine practice of quieting the mind and emotions helps the Therapeutic Touch practitioner to be able to project calm despite being in stressful situations. Health care professionals are also in a position to assess the contribution of Therapeutic Touch to health care, and to explore how best to integrate it into our health care system. The clinical research discussed in earlier chapters point to the usefulness of Therapeutic Touch for pain relief, relief of anxiety, and acceleration of wound healing. More work is needed to contribute to our understanding of its physiological effects on the body, including its effects on the immune system.

In this book we have described some of the research done to determine how Therapeutic Touch affects the body and emotions. For a variety of reasons, Therapeutic Touch is difficult to study. Most medical research evaluates treatments that are uniform for every patient. When physicians study the effects of a drug, for example, each patient receives the same dose of the same medication. In a double-blind, controlled study, neither the physician nor the patient is aware of whether the subject is receiving a drug or placebo. This removes experimenter bias from the outcome and prevents the patients' expectations from affecting the results.

It is impossible to approach Therapeutic Touch experimentation in the same way. The practitioner cannot be separated from the treatment, and is always aware which patients in a research study receive Therapeutic Touch. The treatment also depends on the skill of the practitioner, and the receptivity of the patient. Additionally, the effects of Therapeutic Touch depend to some extent on how long the patient has had the problem. If an illness is chronic, the treatment will accomplish less. Researchers can partially control for these factors by having the same practitioner administer Therapeutic Touch to all patients in the study, and by making sure the practitioners are unaware of the research design. In some studies, the patients are unaware that they are receiving Therapeutic Touch. However, there is always some effect of the treatment that may result simply from human interaction. In the past several years, researchers have attempted to control for this effect by comparing the results of a group receiving Therapeutic Touch with those of another group receiving a mimic treatment.

Despite these challenges to effective research, we continue to gather useful information. One study currently under way is the largest study on Therapeutic Touch to date. Drs. Joan Turner and Ann Clark, of the University of Alabama School of Nursing, are evaluating the use of Therapeutic Touch in treating 150 patients with severe burns. Serious burns destroy the skin, which is one of the body's most important barriers to infection. Burns are also often extremely painful, because nurses and physicians must continually clean the burned area and remove dead skin. Prevention of infection and pain relief are therefore the biggest challenges to the physicians and nurses caring for burn patients.

The University of Alabama study will evaluate patients to

determine if Therapeutic Touch will reduce pain and anxiety in the treated group, and will help treated patients require less pain medication. Researchers postulate that patients receiving Therapeutic Touch will have less pain because the treatments will increase the levels of beta-endorphins in the bloodstream. They will therefore measure endorphin blood levels. Endorphins are the body's natural pain killers. Higher levels of endorphins in the body improve mood and blunt the perception of pain.

Researchers will also determine if the rate of infection is less in the group treated with Therapeutic Touch. They postulate that a lower infection rate will be associated with a greater number of lymphocytes circulating in the patient's blood, and will therefore measure blood lymphocyte levels. These cells determine the body's ability to resist certain kinds of infection. The results of this study, when available, will contribute to our understanding of how Therapeutic Touch exerts its effects.

Not all of the effects of Therapeutic Touch can be dissected in this scientific fashion. To develop a better understanding of how it is effective also requires a different approach. Besides studying the results of Therapeutic Touch experimentally, practitioners can make a contribution to our understanding by evaluating further the *qualitative* experience of both the recipient and practitioner. Rather than simply measuring specific outcomes, such as amount of pain, changes in anxiety, or blood levels of immune cells, researchers need to explore further how Therapeutic Touch contributes to helping people make changes in their lives in ways that promote health. Many recipients of Therapeutic Touch believe that as a result of their treatments the way they choose to live their lives becomes more consistent with their internal sense of self. Patients tell us that they have more energy, are more confident, and feel a connection with an inner self that is not affected by their illness. To collect more information about how and why this is true, and to evaluate *if* it is uniformly true, researchers need to analyze the words and stories of Therapeutic Touch recipients, and allow their life experiences to become evidence for the effectiveness of the technique in helping people to change. In this kind of research, the experience of the patient becomes the focus. In understanding how Therapeutic Touch contributes to the *process* of healing, we explore the whole of a person's experience and its significance to the individual.

A process-oriented approach, which examines life experience, differs from that of modern medicine, where disease and its causes are the focus. In the current scientific worldview, only that which observers can measure is usually considered valid. A broader perspective acknowledges that objective measurement makes a contribution to our understanding, but gives us only part of the truth. By understanding exactly how it is that life changes for recipients of Therapeutic Touch, we increase our understanding of the healing process, and find direction for further study.

Therapeutic Touch is based on a concept of a human being as an open system, always exchanging with others and the environment. From this perspective, an individual is made up of a physical body, emotions, thoughts, and an intuitive self. A person is a dynamic system—our bodies, feelings, and thoughts are always changing. Despite this constant change, there is an orderly relationship and integrated working together of all these aspects of our makeup that defines a state of health. During Therapeutic Touch, the practitioner, with a specific intent to help, uses the fact of energy exchange between individuals to make universal healing energy available to the recipient. This supports the body's inherent tendency toward order. In this way Therapeutic Touch supports the integrated functioning of the whole.

As we mentioned in Chapter Three, this approach to healing is one that is fundamentally different from that of modern medicine. Medical science examines the disease process by reducing it to its component processes and fixing the malfunctioning parts. Because of its reductionistic approach, modern medicine has contributed to an objective understanding of disease and as a result has alleviated suffering. These different approaches to healing need not be mutually exclusive. In fact, as we move into the future and medicine becomes even more high-tech, Therapeutic Touch becomes an important addition to our care of the sick, because it maintains the human connection between practitioner and patient. Health care practitioners can use both the best of medical care, together with Therapeutic Touch as an adjunct, to reduce suffering, relieve pain, and promote healing.

Notes

Chapter 1: Origins

1. Krieger, D. "Therapeutic Touch: Two decades of research, teaching, and clinical practice." *Imprint,* 37 (3). This article originally appeared in the September/October 1990 issue of *Imprint* magazine (the official magazine of the National Student Nurses' Association), pp.86–88.

2. Grad, B., et al. "The influence of an unorthodox method of treatment on wound healing in mice." *Int. Journal of Parapsychology,* 3: 5–24, Spring 1961.

3. Grad, B. "A telekinetic effect on plant growth. Part 2. Experiments involving treatment of saline in stoppered bottles." *Int. Journal of Parapsychology,* 6:473–498, Autumn 1964.

4. Krieger, Dolores. "The response of in-vivo human hemoglobin to an active healing therapy by direct laying on of hands." *Human Dimensions,* 1:12–15, Autumn 1972.

5. Krieger, Dolores. "The relationship of touch, with intent to help or to heal, to subjects' in-vivo hemoglobin values: a study in personalized interaction." *American Nurses' Association Ninth Nursing Research Conference,* held at San Antonio, Texas. March 21–23, 1973. Kansas City, Mo. American Nurses' Association, 1974, pp. 39–58.

6. Krieger, Dolores. "Healing by the laying-on of hands as a facilitator

of bioenergetic exchange: the response of in-vivo human hemoglobin." *Psychoenergetic Systems,* Vol. 3, number 3, 1974.

7. Krieger, Dolores. "Therapeutic touch: The imprimatur of nursing." *American Journal of Nursing,* May 1975, p. 784.

Chapter 2: The Human Energy Field

1. Perrone, B., and H. Stockel and V. Krueger. *Medicine Women, Curanderas, and Women Doctors* (Norman: University of Oklahoma Press, l989), p. 14.

2. Rudhyar, Dane. *The Magic of Tone and the Art of Music* (Boulder: Shambhala Publications, 1982), p. 37.

3. Capra, Fritjof. "The dance of Shiva." *Main Currents in Modern Thought,* Vol. 21, No. 1, 1972.

4. Heisenberg, Werner. *Across the Frontiers* (Woodbridge: Ox Bow Press, 1990), p. 14.

5. Bohm, David. "The implicate order and the super-implicate order." *Dialogues with Scientists and Sages* (London: Routledge & Kegan Paul, 1986), p. 27.

6. Kunz, Fritz. "The reality of the non-material." *Main Currents in Modern Thought,* Vol. 20, No. 2, 1963.

7. Heisenberg, Werner. *Across the Frontiers* (Woodbridge: Ox Bow Press, 1990), p.14.

8. Capra, Fritjof. *The Turning Point* (New York: Bantam Books, 1983), p. 88.

9. Kunz, Fritz. "The reality of the non-material." *Main Currents in Modern Thought,* Vol. 20, No. 2, l963, pp. 34–37.

10. Kunz, Dora, and Erik Peper. "Fields and their clinical implications," *Spiritual Aspects of the Healing Arts* (Wheaton, IL: Theosophical Publishing House, 1985), pp. 213–222.

11. Ibid. p. 222.

Chapter 3: Ideas About Healing

1. Rossi, E. L. *The Psychobiology of Mind-Body Healing.* (New York: W. W. Norton & Co., 1986.)

2. Sheldrake, R. "Morphogenetic fields: nature's habits," in Weber, R., *Dialogues with Scientists and Sages* (London: Routledge & Kegan Paul, 1986), p. 79.

3. Ibid. p. 79.

4. Weber, R. "Philosophical foundations and frameworks for healing," in Kunz, D. (compiler), *Spiritual Aspects of the Healing Arts* (Wheaton, IL.: Theosophical Publishing House, 1985), p. 30.

5. Bohm, D. *Wholeness and the Implicate Order* (London: Routledge & Kegan Paul, 1980), p. 177.

6. Achterberg, J. *Imagery in Healing* (Boston: New Science Library, 1985), p. 101.

7. Braud, W., & M. Schlitz, "Psychokinetic influence on electrodermal activity." *Journal of Parapsychology*, (1983) 47 (2) 95–119.

8. Wilber, K. *The Spectrum of Consciousness* (Wheaton, IL: Theosophical Publishing House, 1977), p. 33.

9. Ibid. p. 33.

10. Johnston, C. M. *The Creative Imperative: A Four-Dimensional Model of Human Growth and Planetary Evolution* (Berkeley: Celestial Arts, 1986), p. 7.

11. Achterberg, op. cit. p. 115.

12. Gruber, B., et al. "Immune system and psychologic changes in metastatic cancer patients while using ritualized relaxation and guided imagery: A pilot study." *Scandinavian Journal of Behavior Therapy*, 17 (1988): 25–46.

13. Achterberg, op. cit. p. 170.

14. Dossey, L. *Healing Words: The Power of Prayer and the Practice of Medicine* (New York: HarperCollins, 1993), p. 241.

Chapter 4: The Method

1. Heidt, Patricia. "Openness: a qualitative analysis of nurses' and patients' experiences of Therapeutic Touch." *IMAGE: Journal of Nursing Scholarship*, Vol. 22 No. 3 (1990), pp. 182–183.

2. Ibid. p. 183.

3. Krieger, Dolores. *Living the Therapeutic Touch* (New York: Dodd, Mead & Company, 1987), p. 33.

4. Macrae, Janet. *Therapeutic Touch, A Practical Guide* (New York: Alfred A. Knopf, 1987), p. 86–87.

Chapter 5: The Effects of Therapeutic Touch

1. Krieger, D. *Accepting Your Power to Heal: The Personal Practice of Therapeutic Touch* (Santa Fe: Bear and Company, Inc., 1993), p. 83.

2. Benson, H., et al. "The relaxation response." *Psychiatry,* 37 (1974) pp. 37–45.

3. Kiecolt-Glaser, J., et al. "Acute psychological stressors and short-term immune changes: What, why, for whom and to what extent," *Psychosomatic Medicine,* 54 (1992) pp. 680–685.

4. Kemeny, Margaret. "Emotions and the immune system," in Moyers, B. *Healing and the Mind* (New York: Doubleday, 1993), p. 201.

5. Pelletier, Kenneth. *Mind as Healer, Mind as Slayer* (New York: Dell, 1992), p. 75.

6. al'Absi, M., et al. "Borderline hypertensives produce exaggerated adrenocortical responses to mental stress." *Psychosomatic Medicine,* 56 (1994) pp. 245–250.

7. Jemmot, J., et al. "Academic stress, power motivation, and decrease in secretion rate of salivary secretion of Ig-A." *Lancet,* 2 (1983) pp. 1400–1414.

8. Kiecolt-Glaser, J., et al. "Chronic stress and immunity in family caregivers of Alzheimer's disease victims." *Psychosomatic Medicine,* 49 (1987) pp. 523–535.

9. Benson, H. op. cit. p. 38.

10. Pelletier, op. cit. pp. 233–235.

11. Rood, Y. R., et al. "The effects of stress and relaxation on the in vitro immune response in man: a meta-analytic study." *Journal of Behavioral Medicine,* 16 (2), pp. 163–81.

12. Krieger, D., et al. "Therapeutic touch: searching for evidence of

physiological change." *American Journal of Nursing,* April 1979, pp. 660–663.

13. Heidt, P. "An investigation of the effect of therapeutic touch on the anxiety of hospitalized patients." Unpublished doctoral thesis, New York University, 1979.

14. Quinn, J. "An Investigation of the effect of therapeutic touch without physical contact on state anxiety of hospitalized cardiovascular patients." Unpublished doctoral thesis, New York University, 1982.

15. Randolph, G. Described in *Nursing Research,* 33 (1) January/February 1984, pp. 33–36.

16. Presented on BBC documentary, "A Way of Healing," TV Ontario's *Vital Signs,* March 23, 1993.

17. Futterman, A., et al. "Immunological and physiological changes associated with induced positive and negative mood." *Psychosomatic Medicine,* 56:499–511 (1994).

18. Pennebaker, J. W., et al. "Disclosure of traumas and immune function: Health implications for psychotherapy." *Journal of Consulting and Clinical Psychology,* 56(2): 239–245 (1988).

19. Keller, E., & V. Bzdek. "Effects of therapeutic touch on tension headache pain." *Nursing Research*, 35(2): 101–106 (1986).

20. Kunz, D., and E. Peper. "The pain process and strategies for pain reduction." *The American Theosophist* (Wheaton, IL: Theosophical Publishing House, 1985), p. 421.

21. Krieger, D. *Accepting Your Power to Heal: The Personal Practice of Therapeutic Touch,* p. 84.

22. Wirth, D. "The effect of noncontact therapeutic touch on the healing rate of full thickness dermal wounds." Master's thesis. JFK University, California, 1989.

Chapter 6: Therapeutic Touch with Children

1. Krieger, D. *Living the Therapeutic Touch* (New York: Dodd, Mead & Co., 1987), p. 157–187.

2. Leduc, E. "The healing touch." *Maternal Child Nursing,* Vol. 14, January 1989, pp. 41–43.

3. Fedoruk, R. "Transfer of the relaxation response: Therapeutic touch as a method of reducing stress in premature neonates." Unpublished Ph.D. dissertation, University of Maryland, 1984.

4. Kramer, N. "Comparison of therapeutic touch and casual touch in stress reduction of hospitalized children." *Pediatric Nursing*, 16:5, pp. 483–85.

Chapter 7: Therapeutic Touch for Serious Illness

1. Michaels, D., and C. Levine. "Estimates of the number of mother-less children orphaned by AIDS in the United States." *Journal of the American Medical Association*, 1992, 268:3456–61.

2. Kunz, D., and E. Peper. "Depression from the energetic perspective: Treatment strategies." *The American Theosophist*, 72 (9) (Wheaton, IL: Theosophical Publishing House, 1984), p. 302.

Chapter 8: Therapeutic Touch for the Dying

1. Solomon, M. Z., et al. "Decisions near the end of life." *American Journal of Public Health*, 1993, 83:14–23.

2. Steinmetz, D., et al. "Family physicians' involvement with dying patients and their families." *Archives of Family Medicine*, 1993, 2:753–761.

Resources

For information about Therapeutic Touch practitioners, teachers, and workshops in the United States:

Nurse Healers Professional Associates, Inc.
P.O. Box 444
Allison Park, Pennsylvania 15101
(412) 355-8476

For information about practitioners, teachers, and workshops in Canada:

The Therapeutic Touch Network
P.O Box 85551
875 Eglinton Avenue West
Toronto, Ontario M6C4A8
(416) 65-TOUCH

For information about invitational Therapeutic Touch workshops for health professionals:

Orcas Island Foundation
Route 1 Box 86
Eastsound, Washington 98245
(360) 376-4526

Pumpkin Hollow Farm
Route 1 Box 135
Craryville, New York 12521
(518) 325-3583

Susan Wager, M.D.

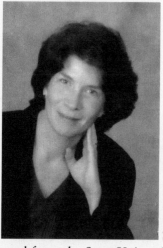

Photo by Jennifer Koski

Dr. Wager graduated from the State University of New York at Stony Brook School of Medicine in 1979, and completed her internship and residency in Internal Medicine at New York University Medical Center in 1982. After completing her medical training she began to study Therapeutic Touch at New York University School of Nursing. Since 1984 Dr. Wager has studied the technique with Dora Kunz, one of its originators.

Since 1985 she has both practiced and taught Therapeutic Touch to health professionals in the Pacific Northwest. In addition, Dr. Wager had a private practice in Internal Medicine in Seattle until 1990.

As a result of her work with Dora Kunz, and her practice of Therapeutic Touch, Dr. Wager developed a special interest in the emotional and mental difficulties that accompany serious illness. She also has an interest in using Therapeutic Touch to help people who are dying. In 1992 she completed an M.A. in Psychology and has recently started a counseling practice.

Dr. Wager lives in Seattle with her husband, also a physician, and their son.

Dora Kunz

In the 1930s Dora Kunz began an association with Dr. Otelia Bengtsson, an allergist in New York City, that initiated a lifelong study of the relationship between emotional patterns and physical disease. Since then she has worked with many physicians, and at their request, observed many famous healers at work. Her study of the healing process led to a collaboration with Dr. Dolores Krieger in 1970, to develop the technique of Therapeutic Touch. For the past fifty years she has continued to refine her understanding of the role that our emotions and habitual thoughts play in promoting illness, and in how they facilitate healing.

Mrs. Kunz is the editor of *Spiritual Aspects of the Healing Arts*, an anthology. She is the author of *The Personal Aura*, and coauthor with Dr. Shafica Karagulla of *The Chakras and the Human Energy Fields*. She is past president of the Theosophical Society in America. Mrs. Kunz now lives in the Pacific Northwest, and travels extensively to teach Therapeutic Touch.